YOUR LABS ARE FINE. YOU'RE NOT.

Understanding the Mineral Deficiencies Your Doctor Can't See

JOY STEPHENSON-LAWS, JD

Edited by Pauline Jose, MD

YOUR LABS ARE FINE. YOU'RE NOT.

Understanding the Mineral Deficiencies Your Doctor Can't See

MEDICAL DISCLAIMER

This book is for informational purposes only and is not intended as a substitute for professional medical advice, diagnosis, or treatment. Always seek the advice of your physician or other qualified health provider with any questions you may have regarding a medical condition. Never disregard professional medical advice or delay in seeking it because of something you have read in this book.

Medical Editor: Pauline Jose, MD

Cover Design: Milan Fritzinger

Published by Proactive Health Labs

www.phlabs.org

ISBN 979–8–9939740–5–7 (Hardback)
ISBN 979–8–9939740–6–4 (Paperback)

First Edition

Printed in the United States of America

10 9 8 7 6 5 4 3 2 1

FOR

Eric

who gave me the space to write,
and stayed patient and present
through all the late nights.

A note before you begin

You're holding this book because something is wrong and no one has been able to tell you what.

You've been to doctors. You've had tests. Everything came back "normal." But you don't feel normal. You feel exhausted, foggy, anxious, achy—like your body is working against you.

I've spent over 40 years as a healthcare attorney, and nearly 15 years as a wellness coach. I've seen this story hundreds of times. People dismissed. People doubted. People told their symptoms are "just stress" or "just aging" when something real is going on.

Your Labs Might Be Fine. But You're Not.

This book is about the gap between "normal" and "optimal"—the place where millions of people suffer without answers. It's about minerals: the nutrients most doctors don't test for, most diets don't provide enough of, and most people have never considered.

I'm not promising minerals are the answer to everything. But for many people, they're a missing piece. That piece might be yours.

One more thing before we begin.

Minerals are a piece of the puzzle. For many people, the missing piece. But not always the whole picture—and not always enough on their own.

If your symptoms are severe, or getting worse, or new—see a doctor. Not instead of reading this book. Alongside it. Some things need medical care this book can't replace, and knowing the difference is part of trusting your body's signal.

The work behind this book didn't start with minerals.

It started with a question: how does the body communicate when something isn't right?

Several of my earlier books explored that question from different angles. In *From Chains to Wings*, I wrote about the patterns our nervous systems run automatically—protectively, often long after the original danger has passed. That work built around a simple practice: notice what's happening, validate it without judgment, then make a small adjustment. Not a dramatic overhaul. Just a small shift from a regulated place.

The workbook that followed made that practice personal, offering exercises and reflection tools for recognizing your own patterns and building awareness of how your body responds to stress.

Secrets That Sparkle (and Secrets That Sting) approached the same idea from another direction. Written as a children's story, it teaches a simple but powerful lesson: not everything that looks fine on the surface actually is. Some things sparkle. Some things sting. And the difference lives in what you feel, not what you're told.

That same principle lives at the heart of this book.

The thread connecting all of these books is the same: **your body is telling you something.** The work—whether you're reading poetry, doing workbook exercises, talking to a child about secrets, or trying to understand why your labs are fine but you're not—is learning to trust that signal.

Start where you are. Not where you think you should be.

— Joy Stephenson-Laws, JD

HOW TO USE THIS BOOK

A reader's guide

This book has four parts:

- **PART I: Mineral Essentials—The Foundation**
- **PART II: Understanding Your Body—When Minerals Aren't Enough**
- **PART III: When Symptoms Speak—What Your Body Is Telling You**
- **PART IV: Making It Work—From Knowledge to Action**

Part I is **WHAT** to do.

Part II is **WHY** it might not be working.

Part III is **WHERE** your symptoms point.

Part IV is **HOW** to make it stick.

You don't have to read them in order. You don't have to read them all. Which parts you need depends on how you're feeling right now.

Do you need medical help right now?

Before we go any further, make sure you don't need immediate care.

Call 911 or Go to an Emergency Room If:

- Chest pain, pressure, or tightness—especially with exertion, or with sweating, nausea, or arm/jaw pain
- Racing or pounding heart that won't stop
- Fainting or nearly fainting
- Severe trouble breathing, or sudden shortness of breath
- Sudden severe headache (worst of your life)
- Sudden face drooping, arm weakness, or slurred speech (signs of stroke)
- Sudden numbness or confusion
- Seizure, or new loss of consciousness
- Coughing or vomiting blood
- Severe abdominal pain that won't ease
- Throat swelling, trouble swallowing, or full-body hives (allergic reaction)

If You're Having Thoughts of Harming Yourself or Others:

Call or text 988 (U.S. Suicide & Crisis Lifeline)

Outside the U.S.: findahelpline.com

See a Doctor This Week If:

- Fatigue so bad you can't work or care for yourself
- Bleeding that won't stop
- Hair falling out in clumps
- Unexplained weight loss (10+ pounds)
- Severe vomiting or diarrhea that won't stop
- Muscle weakness that's getting worse

If none of these apply, this book can help. Keep reading.

Finding your starting point

This book uses a system of three modes:

PROTECTION **SAFETY** **HEALING**

to help you find your starting point and pace yourself appropriately.

Your mode isn't a personality type or a permanent label. It's a description of your capacity right now.

Modes are fluid. You will move between them. That's normal. That's expected. That's your body protecting you.

Go by how you actually feel—not how you think you should feel.

Find your mode

Answer these questions honestly:

- Have you eaten today?
- Do you know what day it is?

If either answer is no—or if reading this page is taking everything you have:

You're in **PROTECTION MODE**. Skip to the Absolute Minimum Protocol below.

If both answers are yes and you can focus, but it's hard:

You're in **SAFETY MODE**. Skip to the Safety Mode section.

If both answers are yes and you feel pretty clearheaded:

You're in **HEALING MODE**. Skip to the Healing Mode section.

> *If you're between modes, start with the gentler option.*

PROTECTION MODE

This book is education, not medical advice—and the doses here are a starting point, not a diagnosis.

"I'm barely functioning."

The Absolute Minimum Protocol (AMP)

You forgot to eat today. You can't remember why you walked into this room. Reading a whole chapter feels impossible. You're in survival mode.

Here's everything you need to do:

Three Foods This Week

- Spinach (frozen is fine)—3–4 times this week. Skip if you take warfarin.
- Canned black beans—rinsed 3–4 times this week
- Pumpkin seeds—daily if possible

One Supplement

- Magnesium glycinate 200 mg at bedtime

That's it. Three foods. One supplement. Nothing else.

Get stable first. Optimize later.

Note: If you take blood thinners (like Warfarin/Coumadin) or have kidney disease, check with your doctor before starting—even this short list.

Your next step: Go to Chapter 3 for complete instructions on how to use these foods.

Check back in 3–4 weeks. If you feel better, turn to Chapter 1. If you feel the same or worse, or if new symptoms show up—see a doctor.

> *If you're in Protection Mode, your path is set. Do the Absolute Minimum Protocol. Go to Chapter 3 for full instructions. That's it for now. The rest of this section is for Safety and Healing Mode readers. You can skip to Chapter 3.*

SAFETY MODE

"I'm stable but struggling."

Signs You're Here

- Functioning, but not thriving
- Some energy for change, but limited
- Able to read, but only in small pieces
- Not in crisis, but not at full strength

Your Path

1. Chapter 1—Figure out if minerals are part of your problem
2. Chapter 2—Learn which tests to ask for
3. Chapter 3—Start with food (the simplest change)
4. Chapter 4—Add supplements only if food isn't enough
5. Part III—Look up your specific symptoms
6. Part II—Read later if you want to understand why

> *Why Part III before Part II? You need practical answers for your symptoms more than theory right now.*

Expect 3–4 weeks for Part I. One thing at a time.

HEALING MODE

"I'm functional and ready to go deeper."

Signs You're Here

- Functioning well day-to-day
- Energy and focus to spare
- Want to understand the "why," not just the "what"
- Ready for real, lasting changes

Your Path

Read all four parts in order. Take your time. Use the checklists fully. Look for patterns.

- Part I gives you tools
- Part II explains why those tools sometimes don't work
- Part III connects your symptoms to specific minerals
- Part IV helps you troubleshoot and maintain your gains

The deeper you go, the more you'll see how everything connects.

Expect 2–3 months for the full journey.

A tool you'll use throughout this book

Feel—Pause—Act is introduced in the Introduction (page iv) and runs throughout this book at key decision points. Before buying supplements, before doctor visits, whenever you're about to take action from an activated state.

Feel

Notice what's happening in your body. Calm? Activated? Overwhelmed?

Pause

Take a breath.
Ask if you're making this decision from a calm place.

Act

Choose one small action from a regulated state—not urgency or fear.

Why this matters:
When your nervous system is in survival mode, your body can't absorb or use nutrients properly. Feel—Pause—Act helps you interrupt that pattern.

> *You'll learn the full practice in Chapter 5, and you'll see it at key decision points—especially before taking action on supplements, testing, or major changes.*

WHAT EVERY CHAPTER CONTAINS

How each chapter is structured

To help you navigate, every chapter follows the same structure:

- **Opening validation**—acknowledging where you might be
- **Core content**—the information you need
- **Practical tools**—scripts, formulas, examples
- **Mode check-in**—next steps for each mode
- **Summary**—what you now know

> *If you get lost, skip to the Mode Check-In at the end of any chapter.*

Ready?

PROTECTION Absolute Minimum Protocol (AMP) + Chapter 3. That's it.

SAFETY Turn to Chapter 1. One step at a time.

HEALING Turn to Chapter 1 and read straight through.

> *Start where you are. That's enough.*

TABLE OF CONTENTS

PART IV: Making It Work—From Knowledge to Action

PART I

Mineral Essentials

The Foundation

In This Section:

- **Chapter 1:** Start Here: Your Mineral Assessment
- **Chapter 2:** Testing + Your First Doctor Visit
- **Chapter 3:** Food First: The Simple Plan
- **Chapter 4:** Supplements: What to Buy (and What to Skip)

CHAPTER 1

Start Here: Your Mineral Assessment

This is the first step everyone takes—figuring out if minerals are actually part of your problem. By the end, you'll know if you should keep reading.

Nobody Took You Seriously (But Your Body Was Right).

You told your doctor something was wrong. Tests came back "normal." They suggested stress management. Better sleep. Maybe an antidepressant.

But here's what I need you to know:

Your body was right. You weren't making it up.

These "normal" test results are built to catch disease, not deficiency. You can have low-normal magnesium, borderline iron, or low-normal zinc—and still feel terrible. Normal isn't optimal.

This chapter helps you figure out if minerals are part of your story. You can skim it in 5 minutes; completing it thoughtfully takes a bit longer.

Before you begin:

If you're having a medical emergency right now, stop and call 911 or 988. (See page VI for full guidance.)

When You Also Need Medical Guidance

This book is for adults who are generally healthy but have mineral deficiencies. Some situations require medical supervision while using this book:

- *Chronic kidney, liver, heart, or lung disease*
- *Had bariatric surgery or intestinal surgery*
- *Take digoxin or 3+ prescription medications*

> - *Genetic conditions affecting mineral processing*
> - *Pregnant, breastfeeding, under 18, or over 75 with multiple health issues*
>
> *This doesn't mean you can't benefit—it means you need your doctor's guidance while using this book. Chapter 2 helps you determine what testing you need.*

Symptom Checklist by Mineral

If you've had the symptom in the past 3 months, check the box. Don't overthink whether it "counts" or if it's "bad enough." If it's happening, check it.

Feeling overwhelmed? If this checklist starts to feel like too much, stop here and go straight to **Chapter 3** for the Absolute Minimum Protocol. You can come back later.

Energy & Fatigue

- [ ] Exhausted most days, even after 7–8 hours of sleep
- [ ] Need multiple cups of coffee just to function
- [ ] Hit a wall around 2–3 PM every day
- [ ] Can barely get through workouts or avoid them entirely
- [ ] Feel more tired than you did 6 months ago

If you checked ***3+****: Often low in* ***iron*** *or* ***magnesium***

Muscles & Movement

- [ ] Muscle cramps, especially at night in legs
- [ ] Restless legs when trying to sleep
- [ ] Muscle twitches for no reason
- [ ] Unexplained weakness
- [ ] Very sore muscles for days after minor exercise

*If you checked **3+**: Often low in **magnesium** or **potassium***

Brain & Mood

- [ ] Can't focus or concentrate like before
- [ ] Forget words or why you entered a room
- [ ] Feel anxious or irritable more than usual
- [ ] PMS mood swings (women)
- [ ] Feel down or depressed without clear reason

*If you checked **3+**: May be low in **magnesium**, **zinc**, or **iron***

Heart & Blood Pressure

- [ ] Blood pressure 130/80 or higher
- [ ] Heart skips beats or races
- [ ] Dizzy when standing up quickly
- [ ] Been told your blood pressure is a concern

*If you checked **2+**: Often low in **magnesium** or **potassium***

Immune & Healing

- [ ] Catch every cold that goes around
- [ ] Cuts and scrapes heal slowly
- [ ] Sick more than 3 times per year
- [ ] Feel like immune system is weak

*If you checked **2+**: Often low in **zinc** or **selenium***

Hair, Skin & Nails

- [ ] Hair falling out more than usual
- [ ] Nails brittle and break easily
- [ ] Dry skin or skin problems
- [ ] White spots on nails

*If you checked **2+**: Often low in **iron**, **zinc**, or **selenium***

Sleep

- [ ] Can't fall asleep easily
- [ ] Wake up multiple times per night
- [ ] Wake up feeling unrefreshed
- [ ] Legs won't let you relax at bedtime

*If you checked **2+**: Often low in **magnesium** or **iron***

Digestion

- [ ] Constipated frequently
- [ ] Chronic diarrhea
- [ ] Bloated after meals
- [ ] Diagnosed with IBD (Crohn's, colitis)

*If you checked **2+**: Gut issues can block absorption—**testing recommended***

Women Only

- [ ] Terrible PMS (cramps, mood, bloating)
- [ ] Very heavy periods
- [ ] Menopausal symptoms

*If you checked **2+**: Often low in **magnesium**, **calcium**, or **iron***

Men Only

- [ ] Low energy or reduced motivation
- [ ] Decreased muscle mass or strength
- [ ] Low libido or sex drive
- [ ] Erectile dysfunction
- [ ] Male pattern baldness (more than typical)
- [ ] Fertility concerns

*If you checked **2+**: May be low in **zinc**, **selenium**, or **magnesium***

Pain

- [ ] Chronic pain
- [ ] Frequent migraines or headaches
- [ ] Diagnosed with fibromyalgia or widespread pain

*If you checked **2+**: Often low in **magnesium***

Other Symptoms

- ☐ Cold hands and feet all the time
- ☐ Loss of taste or smell
- ☐ Cracks at corners of mouth

*If you checked 1+: Often low in **iron** (cold extremities), **zinc** (taste/smell), or **iron/B vitamins** (mouth cracks)*

Your Total Score

Count your total checkmarks across ALL sections above.

☐ Checkmarks

These ranges aren't diagnostic—they're practical groupings to guide your next steps. A high score doesn't mean every symptom is mineral-related; it means minerals are likely part of the picture.

What to Do Next

Now that you have a score, use the guidance below to determine your next step. Find your current mode first, then look at the recommendations for your score range. *(Not sure which mode you're in? See "Find Your Mode" in the first section, or simply ask: Can I focus right now? If barely, you're in Protection Mode.)*

PROTECTION MODE

It doesn't matter what your score is.

Go to Chapter 3 for the Absolute Minimum Protocol (AMP). Stabilize first, optimize later.

Come back to these chapters when you're functioning better.

SAFETY MODE

Look at your total score and find yourself below:

Low Score (0–10 checkmarks)

Minimal symptoms, decent diet. Likely getting adequate minerals with room to improve.

Your next step:

Chapter 3 (Food First). That's it. Pick 2–3 mineral-rich foods and start eating them regularly. No supplements or testing needed yet.

Medium Score (11–20 checkmarks)

Real symptoms. Not imaginary, not "just stress." Probably 1–2 mineral deficiencies.

Your next steps:

This week: Chapter 3 (Food First) + Chapter 2 (Testing)

Next month: Chapter 4 (Supplements) if food alone isn't enough after 2–3 weeks

Give this 8–12 weeks to work.

High Score (21+ checkmarks)

A lot going on. Multiple symptoms. Very likely several mineral deficiencies are contributing. This isn't your fault.

Your next steps:

This week: All of Part I (Chapters 1–4) + Call your doctor for comprehensive mineral testing

This month: Start 2–3 targeted supplements based on test results

Don't wait to start eating better—do that now.

HEALING MODE

You can handle comprehensive protocols regardless of your score. You want to understand mechanisms, not just follow instructions.

Your path:

This week: Read all of Part I. Complete all assessments thoroughly—analyze the patterns. Request comprehensive mineral testing.

This month: Get tested and understand what the numbers mean. Read Part II to understand nervous system and gut connections. Develop a strategic supplementation plan.

You've Finished Chapter 1

Take a breath. Here's what you know now:

- ✓ Whether minerals are likely part of your problem
- ✓ Which minerals you're probably low in
- ✓ Your next specific step

Feeling stable? *Turn to your next assigned chapter.*

Feeling overwhelmed? You may have dropped into Protection Mode. That's okay. Go to Chapter 3 for the Absolute Minimum Protocol.

Minerals matter, but they're not magic.

Improvements take 6–12 weeks minimum.

You don't have to be perfect—you just have to take the next right step.

You've taken the first step. That's huge.

CHAPTER 2

Testing + Your First Doctor Visit

Not everyone needs testing. But everyone benefits from understanding what tests mean and when they matter.

You Shouldn't Have to Fight This Hard

You just want to know what's going on in your own body. That shouldn't be controversial. But somehow, asking for a simple blood test can feel like preparing for battle.

The system wasn't designed to make this easy. Insurance doesn't always cover mineral testing. Doctors have 15 minutes per patient and a checklist that doesn't include"check for nutritional deficiencies." Many were never taught that sub-clinical deficiencies exist—or that they matter.

Wanting to understand your own lab results isn't obsessive. It's informed. This chapter gives you the tools to navigate that system—whether that means working with your doctor, working around them, or doing it yourself.

Feeling overwhelmed?
If this chapter starts to feel like too much, stop here and go to **Chapter 3** for the Absolute Minimum Protocol. You can come back to testing later.

Do You Actually Need Testing?

Testing can tell you exactly which minerals you're low in and how low you are. But here's what most people don't realize: **you might not need testing at all.**

Testing is useful. But it's not always necessary. And it's rarely the first step.

First Question: Have You Tried Food Yet?

Have you made mineral-rich food changes for 6–8 weeks?

No → Skip testing for now. Go to Chapter 3, make the food changes, then comeback in eight weeks. Testing before you've tried food is premature.

Yes, and I feel better → Skip testing. Keep doing what's working. You don't need numbers to validate improvement.

Yes, and nothing changed → Keep reading. You likely need testing.

If You're Generally Healthy

No chronic conditions. You eat a varied diet with whole foods. Not on any medications. You feel pretty good and just want to "optimize."

Skip testing. You're probably fine. Spend your time and energy on eating good food, not chasing lab numbers.

The Testing Decision Checklist

This checklist tells you whether to test—and how urgently.

Section A1: Immediate Testing Required

If you check even one of these, schedule testing this week. These situations can create dangerous mineral imbalances.

- ☐ I take digoxin
- ☐ I have chronic kidney disease
- ☐ I had bariatric surgery (gastric bypass, sleeve, etc.)
- ☐ I have severe symptoms that disrupt my ability to function

IF YOU CHECKED ANY BOX ABOVE:
Stop here. You need testing. Schedule it this week.

Section A2: Testing Strongly Recommended

These situations commonly lead to mineral imbalances. Testing is strongly recommended, though not as urgent as A1.

- [ ] I'm on long-term diuretics (water pills like HCTZ, Lasix, Chlorthalidone)
- [ ] I've been on PPIs (Prilosec, Nexium, Prevacid, Protonix) for more than a year

If you checked either box: *Schedule testing within the next few weeks. Don't ignore this, but it's not an emergency.*

Section B: Medications That Can Deplete Minerals

These medications are associated with mineral depletion over time.

- [ ] ACE Inhibitors (drugs ending in "-pril" like lisinopril, enalapril)
  → can deplete zinc
- [ ] H2 blockers (Pepcid, Zantac)
  → can deplete iron and B12
- [ ] Antacids daily (Tums, Rolaids)
  → can deplete magnesium and phosphorus
- [ ] Metformin
  → can deplete B12, possibly magnesium
- [ ] Daily NSAIDs (Advil, Aleve, ibuprofen, naproxen)
  → can cause slow iron loss
- [ ] Corticosteroids (prednisone)
  → can deplete calcium, potassium, and magnesium
- [ ] Birth control pills
  → can deplete magnesium and possibly B vitamins

Section C: High-Risk Conditions and Life Situations

Medical Conditions

- [ ] Crohn's, celiac, or ulcerative colitis
- [ ] Type 2 diabetes or prediabetes
- [ ] Autoimmune disease
- [ ] Chronic digestive issues

Life Stage

- [ ] Pregnant or trying to conceive
- [ ] Breastfeeding
- [ ] Menopausal or perimenopausal
- [ ] Age 65 or older

Women's Health

- [ ] Very heavy periods
- [ ] Donate blood regularly

Lifestyle

- [ ] Endurance athlete
- [ ] Vegetarian or vegan
- [ ] Very low-calorie diet (under 1,200 calories)

Section D: Persistent Symptoms Despite Diet Changes

- ☐ I made diet changes for 2–3 months and my symptoms are still here
- ☐ I have chronic symptoms that disrupt my life—fatigue, cramps, brain fog, hair loss
- ☐ I tried the Absolute Minimum Protocol and saw no improvement

Your Checkmark Counts

Section A1	Section A2	Section B	Section C	Section D	**Total (B + C + D only)**
☐	☐	☐	☐	☐	☐

What Your Score Means

Any checkmarks in Section A1

Testing is urgent. Schedule it this week. These situations can create dangerous mineral imbalances.

Any checkmarks in Section A2

Testing is strongly recommended. Schedule it within the next few weeks.

3+ total checkmarks (Sections B, C, or D)

Testing is recommended. Your situation makes deficiency likely. You need to know what you're dealing with so you're not just guessing.

1–2 total checkmarks (Sections B, C, or D)

Testing is optional but helpful. Consider it if you have the resources and want clarity.

0 checkmarks

Skip testing for now. You're generally healthy with no major risk factors. Spend your time on eating good food. Come back if symptoms develop or persist.

The Five Tests Worth Getting

Most mineral tests are either unreliable or unnecessary. These five actually provide useful information.

One thing to know before you read these: the targets in this chapter are wellness targets, not clinical thresholds. They reflect where research suggests you need to be to feel well—not just avoid disease. Your doctor may use different reference ranges. Both can be right at the same time.

Quick Reference: Do I Need This Test?

Test	Who Benefits Most	Skip If
RBC Magnesium	Cramps, insomnia, anxiety, migraines	Asymptomatic with good diet
Iron Panel	Fatigue, hair loss, heavy periods, vegetarians	Recent normal labs
Vitamin D	Low sun exposure, darker skin, indoor workers	Recent normal test
Zinc	Frequent colds, slow healing, skin/hair issues	Asymptomatic
Potassium	On diuretics, BP meds, muscle cramps	Already in standard bloodwork (Comprehensive Metabolic Panel (CMP))

Test #1: RBC Magnesium (Not Serum Magnesium)

RBC stands for "red blood cell." This is the one that actually matters.

Serum magnesium—the standard test your doctor usually orders—catches severe deficiency but misses the early stages. That's because your body borrows magnesium from your bones and cells to keep your blood levels looking normal. By the time your blood test flags a problem, your tissues have already been running low for a while.

RBC magnesium measures what's inside your red blood cells, where magnesium actually does its work.

Get this test if you have: *muscle cramps, insomnia, anxiety, migraines, or high blood pressure.*

What you're looking for: Middle to top third of the reference range. If you're in the bottom third and you have symptoms, you're functionally deficient—even if the lab calls it "normal."

Test #2: Complete Iron Panel

Don't just test one thing. You need all three pieces:

- **Ferritin**—your iron reserves (how much you have stored)
- **Serum iron**—iron in your blood right now
- **TIBC**—how well your body transports iron

You can have normal iron levels but depleted ferritin. Or normal ferritin but poor iron transport. You need the complete picture.

Get this test if you have: *chronic fatigue or hair loss. Women and vegetarians benefit from routine testing*

What you're looking for:

Ferritin: 50–100 ng/mL for women, 100–200 ng/mL for men (Not the lab's reference range, typically 12–150 ng/mL for women, 12–300 ng/mL for men)

Serum iron: 60–170 mcg/dL

TIBC: 250–450 mcg/dL

These are functional targets used by many clinicians. Your doctor may use different reference ranges.

Below 30 for women or 50 for men? You'll often have symptoms even though you're not technically anemic yet.

Test #3: Vitamin D

Yes, this isn't technically a mineral. But it's essential for calcium absorption and mineral metabolism. Studies estimate about 40% of Americans have insufficient vitamin D levels. For most people, food alone doesn't provide enough. Sun exposure is also unreliable—sunscreen blocks synthesis, winter limits UVB, many people work indoors, and darker skin requires more exposure.

Because of this, vitamin D testing is worth it for anyone who fits those risk factors.

What you're looking for: 40–60 ng/mL. Not just "in range" at 20–30. Actually in the middle-to-upper part of the range.

Test #4: Serum Zinc

Zinc is critical for immune function, wound healing, hormones, skin health, taste and smell, and reproductive health.

Low zinc is associated with frequent colds, hair loss, acne, slow wound healing, and can affect testosterone levels in men.

Get this test if you have: *frequent colds, slow wound healing, hair loss, acne, loss of taste or smell, or hormonal issues.*

What you're looking for: 90–120 mcg/dL

Test #5: Serum Potassium

Good news: This is already included in standard bloodwork. It's part of the basic metabolic panel your doctor orders all the time.

Worth noting: Most doctors only look at whether you're in range, not where you fall in that range.

Potassium is critical for heart rhythm, muscle function, and blood pressure regulation. Even within "normal" range, being on the low end can cause symptoms.

Important for: *Everyone, especially people on diuretics (water pills).*

What you're looking for: 4.0–4.5 mEq/L. Not just "in range" (3.5–5.0), but actually in the middle-to-upper part.

How to Read Your Results: The Rule of Thirds

You get your test results back. Nothing is flagged. Your doctor says "Everything looks normal."But you still feel terrible.

The Problem With "Normal"

Labs set their ranges based on what's average for everyone—not what you need to feel good. Labs are designed to catch dangerous levels, not the suboptimal ones that cause symptoms.

The Rule of Thirds

Forget "normal" or "abnormal." Use this instead:
This is a practical framework, not a diagnostic standard. It's meant to guide next steps, not replace clinical judgment.

Bottom Third	Middle Third	Top Third
With symptoms = functionally deficient	No symptoms = adequate With symptoms = borderline	Optimal—where you want to be

If you're in the bottom third with symptoms:

You're functionally deficient even if the lab says "normal."

What to do: Start supplementing. Increase food sources. Retest in three months.

If you're in the middle third with no symptoms:

You're adequate. Your levels are fine.

What to do: Keep eating well. No supplements needed.

If you're in the middle third with symptoms:

You're borderline. It's worth trying supplementation.

What to do: Try targeted supplementation for two months and track symptoms. If nothing changes, minerals may not be the primary driver.

If you're in the top third:

You're optimal. This is where you want to be.

What to do: Maintain your current intake through food and/or supplements.

> **Example: What This Looks Like With Real Numbers**
>
> ***Your result:*** *Magnesium 1.8 mg/dL*
>
> ***Reference range:*** *1.7–2.2*
>
> ***Doctor says:*** *"Normal."*
>
> ***What's happening:*** *You're in the bottom 20%. Muscle cramps four nights/week. Insomnia. Only getting 180 mg magnesium daily (45% of RDA).*
>
> ***Reality:*** *You're functionally deficient.*
>
> ***Action:*** *Start magnesium glycinate 400 mg at bedtime. Add spinach, pumpkin seeds, almonds. Retest in three months. Goal: 2.0–2.2.*

When Results Are Dangerous (Not Just Suboptimal)

Most mineral imbalances are uncomfortable but not dangerous. But some can be life-threatening.

Call your doctor immediately if your results show:

Potassium very high (>5.5) or very low (<3.0)
Can cause fatal heart arrhythmias. Your heart needs potassium in a very narrow range.

Calcium very high (>10.5) or very low (<8.5)
Can cause kidney stones, severe confusion, seizures, and heart rhythm problems.

Sodium very low (<130) or very high (>150)
Can cause brain swelling, seizures, and severe confusion.

Magnesium very high (>2.5) if you have kidney disease
Can cause breathing problems and cardiac arrest if kidneys can't clear excess.

Feel—Pause—Act: Before Your Doctor Visit

Doctor appointments can be activating—especially when you're asking for something outside the usual script. Before you go in, check in with yourself.

Feel

What's happening in your body right now? Are you anxious about being dismissed? Frustrated from past experiences? Rehearsing arguments in your head?

Pause

Take a breath. You're not walking into a fight—you're asking a professional for a service. You have a right to request testing. Your doctor isn't the enemy.

Act

Go in prepared but calm. Use the scripts below. If they say no, you have options. This isn't your only chance.

Working with Your Doctor

Most doctors genuinely want to help. But they're working within a system that gives them 15 minutes per patient and doesn't reimburse for nutrition counseling. That means you need to approach this strategically.

What to Prepare Before Your Appointment

1. Document your symptoms

Write this down and bring it. Include: What (specific symptoms), When (when they started), How often, Severity (1–10), Impact (how they affect daily life).

> *"I've had calf cramps 4–5 nights per week for three months. Severity 7 out of 10. They wake me up and I'm exhausted the next day, which is affecting my work performance."*

Compare to: "I just feel really tired and my legs hurt sometimes."—vague and easy to dismiss.

2. List all your medications

All prescription medications, OTC medications (including daily ibuprofen, Tums, allergy meds), and all supplements. Some medications deplete minerals—your doctor needs the full picture.

3. Write down exactly what you want

Don't just hope your doctor will think of it. Be specific about what you're asking for.

What to Say in the First 30 Seconds

This is critical. You need to set the tone immediately.

> *"I know we only have 15 minutes, so I'll be specific. I've had [symptoms] for [timeframe]. I've made diet changes for [weeks/months] and tracked my intake—I'm only getting [X] mg of [mineral] daily, which is [%] of the RDA. Based on my symptoms and low dietary intake, I'd like to test for mineral deficiencies before we try other treatments. Specifically, I'd like RBC magnesium, a complete iron panel, and zinc added to my next bloodwork."*

Why this works: You show you're informed and prepared. You tried food first. You present data, not just feelings. You make a specific, reasonable request. You frame it as collaborative.

When Your Doctor Pushes Back

Doctor says: "These tests aren't medically necessary."

You say: "I've had these symptoms for three months now. I want to rule out deficiencies before we try other treatments. If insurance won't cover it, I'm happy to pay out of pocket."

Doctor says: "If you were deficient, you'd be really sick."

You say: "I understand severe deficiency causes serious disease. But low levels that aren't dangerous yet can still cause symptoms. I want to see where I fall in the reference range, not just whether I'm flagged as abnormal."

Doctor says: "Let's try [medication] first."

You say: "I'm open to that if we determine it's necessary. Can we run these tests at the same time so we have baseline data before starting medication? That way we'll know if the medication is what's helping or if it was a deficiency all along."

If They Still Say No

You have three options:

Option 1: Ask for it in writing

"I understand you don't think testing is necessary. Can you document in my chart that I requested RBC magnesium, ferritin, and zinc testing, and that you declined?"

Why it works: Doctors don't like documenting refusal. Many will order the tests rather than write down that they said no.

Option 2: Offer to pay out of pocket

"If insurance won't cover it, I'm willing to pay cash for the testing. Can you still order it?"

Option 3: Order tests yourself

See the next section. You don't actually need your doctor's permission.

How to Order Tests Yourself

You don't need your doctor's permission to get lab testing. Several companies let you order your own bloodwork online. Depending on the lab and panel, most people spend roughly $50–$300 out of pocket.

Services That Let You Order Your Own Tests

- **Quest Direct** and **Labcorp On Demand** work in most states
- **Ulta Lab Tests** or **Walk-In Lab** let you order online and go to whichever lab is closest

How It Works

1. Go to the website and order the tests you want
2. Get a requisition form emailed to you
3. Go to your local Quest or Labcorp location
4. Get your blood drawn—takes about five minutes
5. Results emailed to you in 2–5 days

Important Things to Know

- **Not all states allow this.** New York, New Jersey, and Rhode Island have restrictions.
- **Some tests require fasting.** The website will tell you.
- **Results come with reference ranges but no interpretation.** Use the "Rule of Thirds" to understand your numbers.
- **You can bring results to any doctor**—or a functional medicine practitioner—for interpretation.

Protection—Safety—Healing Check-in

You just learned about testing. Before you move on, check in with yourself.

Are you overwhelmed?

1. Go to the website and order the tests you want
2. Get a requisition form emailed to you
3. Go to your local Quest or Labcorp location
4. Get your blood drawn—takes about five minutes
5. Results emailed to you in 2–5 days

Too much information? Feeling stressed about this? You're in Protection mode—or you dropped into it during this chapter.

Here's what to do: Stop reading. You don't need to figure out testing right now. Go to Chapter 3. Do the Absolute Minimum Protocol. Testing isn't urgent. Stabilizing is urgent.

Are you stable?

Have some clarity about whether you need testing? You're in Safety mode.

Pick one action this week:

- Call your doctor's office to request testing, OR
- Order tests yourself online, OR
- Skip testing and go straight to Chapter 3 (Food First)

Just one action. Not all three.

Are you engaged and ready to be strategic?

You're in Healing mode. Decide your testing strategy:

- Will you work with your regular doctor?
- Do you need to find a functional medicine provider?
- Or will you order tests yourself to maintain control?

Make your plan. Execute it. Then move to Chapter 3 while you wait for results. Don't sit around waiting—start eating better now.

You've Finished Chapter 2

You now understand:

- ✔ Whether you actually need testing
- ✔ Which tests matter (and which don't)
- ✔ How to read results beyond "normal"
- ✔ How to work with your doctor (or work around them)
- ✔ Your options if you can't get what you need

Your next step:

If you're getting tested: Schedule it, then move to Chapter 3. Don't wait for results to start eating better.

If you're skipping testing: Go directly to Chapter 3 (Food First).

Either way, Chapter 3 is next.
Everyone benefits from the food foundation.

CHAPTER 3

Food First: The Simple Plan

Everyone starts here. Whether you're testing or not. Whether you're supplementing or not. Food is your foundation.

You don't need to read this all at once. Skim the sections that match your capacity. If you're barely functioning, skip straight to ***The Absolute Minimum Protocol (AMP)*** below.

You've Heard All This Before

Eat more vegetables. Cut the junk. You know the drill.

But here's what nobody tells you: Knowing what to eat and actually doing it when you're exhausted, overwhelmed, and barely holding things together are two completely different things.

This chapter isn't about perfection. It's not about cutting anything out. It's about adding a few specific foods that will give you the minerals you're missing—without overhauling your entire life.

If you can add three things to what you're already eating, you're doing enough.

Barely functioning right now? Skip ahead to ***The Absolute Minimum Protocol (AMP)*** below. Three foods, one supplement. That's all you need this week.

Why Food Beats Pills (The 30-Second Truth)

A spinach salad with beans, pumpkin seeds, and salmon gives you:

- Magnesium, iron, zinc, calcium, potassium
- Protein, fiber, omega-3 fatty acids
- B vitamins, antioxidants
- Hundreds of compounds we haven't even discovered yet—all working together

A handful of pills gives you:

- Isolated minerals
- Nothing else
- A higher risk of creating imbalances if you guess wrong about what you need

You need both sometimes. But always start with food.

You Don't Have to Be Perfect (Just Start)

You don't have to overhaul your entire diet overnight. In fact, please don't. That's how people burn out and quit within 3 weeks.

Here's what actually works:

Week 1

Add one of the Magnificent Seven foods you don't currently eat.
Just one.

Week 2

Add one more.

Week 3

Try one of the simple meal formulas.

Week 4

Add one more food.

That's it. Four small changes in a month. By the end of 3 months, you've made 12 small changes. Your diet is transformed. And you didn't white-knuckle your way through some restrictive plan you hated every day.

You're not starting a diet. You're adding nutrients. Big difference.

What "Food First" Doesn't Mean

DOESN'T MEAN

"Food only." If you're severely deficient, you need supplements while you improve your diet. Food maintains levels. Supplements correct deficiencies. Both have a place.

DOESN'T MEAN

"Perfect eating." You can eat fast food occasionally, have dessert, drink coffee, enjoy a beer. The goal isn't purity—it's getting enough minerals most days.

DOESN'T MEAN

"Expensive organic everything." Frozen vegetables have the same minerals as fresh. Canned beans work just as well. Store-brand oats are nutritionally identical to fancy ones.

DOESN'T MEAN

"Cooking from scratch every meal." Pre-washed greens, rotisserie chicken, canned beans, frozen brown rice—all of these count. Shortcuts are fine.

DOES MEAN

Make mineral-rich foods the foundation of what you eat, most of the time. That's the bar.

The Magnificent Seven Foods

These seven food categories cover most of the minerals people are commonly missing. Eat all seven every week—not every day, just sometime during the week—and you're likely covered.

You don't need to memorize the numbers below. They're here to show why these foods matter.

Dark Leafy Greens

Spinach, kale, collard greens, Swiss chard, bok choy

WHAT THEY GIVE YOU

½ cup cooked spinach: 78 mg magnesium, 3.2 mg iron, 420 mg potassium

1 cup cooked kale: 94 mg calcium

How much: 1–2 cups cooked (or 2–3 cups raw) at least 4 times per week

If you hate salad: Wilt spinach into scrambled eggs. Blend kale into smoothies. Sauté bok choy in stir-fries. Add Swiss chard to soup. Fresh, frozen, cooked, raw—they all give you minerals.

Beans and Lentils

Black beans, kidney beans, chickpeas, lentils, white beans

WHAT THEY GIVE YOU

½ cup cooked: ~3.3 mg iron, 60 mg magnesium, 305–595 mg potassium, 1–2 mg zinc

How much: 1 cup cooked, 4–5 times per week

If you don't know how to cook beans: Buy them canned. Drain, rinse (removes ~40% sodium), add to anything—salads, soups, rice bowls, tacos, pasta.

If beans make you gassy: Start with lentils—they're easier to digest. Work up to other beans slowly.

Nuts and Seeds

Almonds, cashews, pumpkin seeds, sunflower seeds, Brazil nuts

WHAT THEY GIVE YOU

1 oz (small handful): 80–156 mg magnesium depending on type

Pumpkin seeds: 2.2 mg zinc per ounce

Most nuts/seeds: 1–2 mg iron

Brazil nuts are one of the richest sources of selenium—1–2 nuts often covers your daily needs, though selenium content varies widely depending on where they were grown.

How much: 1 ounce (small handful) daily

Easy ways to add them: Pumpkin seeds on salad. Almond butter in oatmeal. Handful of cashews mid-afternoon. Sunflower seeds in yogurt.

If you have nut allergies: Seeds work just as well—pumpkin, sunflower, chia, flax.

Whole Grains

Brown rice, quinoa, oats, whole wheat bread

WHAT THEY GIVE YOU

1 serving: 42–86 mg magnesium, 1–2 mg iron, 1–2 mg zinc

How much: 3–4 servings daily (1 serving = 1 cup cooked rice/quinoa/oatmeal, or 2 slices whole wheat bread)

If you're used to white rice: Switch gradually. Do half brown, half white for a few weeks. Your taste buds will adjust.

Potatoes (With the Skin—Critical)

Sweet potatoes, regular potatoes, red potatoes

WHAT THEY GIVE YOU

1 medium baked potato with skin: 941 mg potassium (highest common food source)

1 medium sweet potato: 48 mg magnesium + some iron

How much: 1 medium potato, 4–5 times per week

Don't peel them—the skin is where much of the fiber and minerals are. Scrub them clean and eat the whole thing. Bake them, roast cubes with olive oil, add to soup, make oven wedges.

Yogurt and Dairy (Or Fortified Plant Milk)

Plain yogurt, milk, cheese, cottage cheese—or fortified plant milk

WHAT THEY GIVE YOU

1 serving (1 cup yogurt/milk, or ~1 oz cheese): 300–450 mg calcium, 300–400 mg potassium, 1–2 mg zinc

How much: 2–3 servings daily

If you're lactose intolerant: Lactose-free milk exists. Greek yogurt has less lactose. Hard cheeses (cheddar) have almost none.

If you're vegan: Look for plant milks fortified with calcium and vitamin D. Check the label—not all are fortified.

Meat, Fish, or Protein Alternatives

Red meat, poultry, fish, tofu, tempeh, eggs

WHAT THEY GIVE YOU

4–6 oz serving: 3–5 mg iron (best-absorbed type), 3–7 mg zinc, 30–60 mcg selenium

How much: 4–6 oz, 4–5 times per week

Why animal protein matters for iron: Heme iron (from meat) absorbs roughly 2 to 3 times better than plant iron

If you don't eat meat: Tofu, tempeh, and eggs still provide some minerals, but pay extra attention to iron. Pair plant-based iron with vitamin C to increase absorption.

Eat all seven categories every week, and you're covering most of your mineral needs without thinking too hard about it.

Quick check-in:

✎ Which 2–3 of these seven do you already eat regularly? (Mental note or jot them down.)

✎ Which one could you add this week?

Power Foods (Optional Extra Credit)

A few foods are so mineral-dense they deserve mention. You don't need these—the Magnificent Seven are enough. But if one sounds appealing, add it.

OYSTERS

3 oz = 74 mg zinc (a week's worth). If you like them, eat them.

PUMPKIN SEEDS

1 oz = 156 mg magnesium + 2.2 mg zinc. Throw them on everything.

DARK CHOCOLATE (70%+)

1 oz (3–4 squares) = 64 mg magnesium. Not the whole bar.

SARDINES (WITH BONES)

3 oz can = 325 mg calcium (more than milk) +omega-3s. Eat 2–3x/week.

Note: Brazil nuts (selenium) and black strap molasses (iron) are also mineral-dense if you want to explore further.

Simple Meal Formulas

Instead of specific recipes, here are formulas. Once you understand the pattern, you can make hundreds of different meals. You're not following recipes—you're picking ingredients from categories.

Formula #1: The Power Bowl

10 minutes

Quick version: Grain + protein + vegetables + seeds + simple dressing.

BASE (PICK ONE)

Cooked rice | Quinoa | Couscous

PROTEIN (PICK ONE)

1 cup beans (canned) | 2 scrambled eggs | 4 oz tofu, cubed

VEGETABLES (2 CUPS OF WHATEVER YOU HAVE)

Spinach | Raw broccoli | Tomatoes | Avocado | Shredded carrots

CRUNCH (2 TBSP)

Pumpkin seeds | Sunflower seeds | Chopped almonds

DRESSING (PICK ONE)

Olive oil + lemon + salt | Tahini + water + garlic | Soy sauce + rice vinegar + ginger

How to Make It

Put base in bowl. Add protein. Add vegetables. Sprinkle crunch. Drizzle dressing. Eat.

What you get: 200+ mg magnesium, 5+ mg iron, 3+ mg zinc

Formula #2: The Sheet Pan Dinner

5 minutes prep, 30 minutes baking

Quick version: Protein + cubed potato + vegetables, all on one pan, olive oil, 425°F.

PROTEIN (4–6 OZ, PICK ONE)

Chicken breast/thighs | Salmon fillet | Pork chop | Firm tofu

STARCH

1 large potato with skin, cubed

VEGETABLES (2 CUPS)

Broccoli florets | Brussels sprouts | Bell peppers | Red onion

How to Make It

Toss everything with olive oil, salt, pepper, garlic. Spread on sheet pan in single layer. Bake at 425°F for 25–30 minutes. The oven does all the work.

What you get: 150+ mg magnesium, 4+ mg iron, 4+ mg zinc, 1,000+ mg potassium

Formula #3: The Loaded Salad

8 minutes

Quick version: Big bowl of greens + protein + colorful vegetables + nuts/seeds + olive oil dressing.

GREENS (2–3 CUPS)

Spinach | Kale (chopped) | Mixed greens

PROTEIN (PICK ONE)

1 can sardines/tuna | 2 hard-boiled eggs | 1 cup chickpeas | 4 oz leftover chicken

VEGETABLES (3–4 TYPES)

Cherry tomatoes | Cucumber | Bell peppers | Shredded carrots | Red onion

CRUNCH (2 TBSP NUTS OR SEEDS)

DRESSING

Olive oil + vinegar + lemon + salt

How to Make It

Put greens in big bowl. Add everything else. Pour dressing. Toss. Eat.

What you get: 150+ mg magnesium, 6+ mg iron, 4+ mg zinc

Sample Days: Three Different Approaches

You don't need a rigid meal plan. You just need to see what this actually looks like in real life. Pick the one that fits your actual lifestyle.

Sample Day #1: The Busy Person Using Shortcuts

For people who don't have time or energy for elaborate cooking. Everything here is fast and requires minimal skill.

BREAKFAST

Oatmeal + peanut butter + banana (5 minutes)

Cook ½ cup oats in microwave. Stir in 2 tbsp peanut butter. Top with sliced banana.

LUNCH

Rotisserie chicken + pre-washed greens + canned chickpeas (3 minutes)

Pull chicken off store-bought rotisserie. Toss with pre-washed greens and rinsed chickpeas. Drizzle olive oil and lemon.

DINNER

Sheet pan salmon + potato + broccoli (5 minutes prep, 30 minutes baking)

Salmon fillet, cubed potato with skin, broccoli florets on sheet pan. Olive oil, salt, pepper. Bake 425°F for 30 minutes.

What This Day Covers

All seven Magnificent Seven categories. Protein at every meal. Minimal active cooking time.

Magnesium	300+ mg	Iron	12+ mg
Zinc	8+ mg	Calcium	600+ mg
Potassium	2,800+ mg		

Sample Day #2: The Vegetarian

For people who don't eat meat. You need to be more strategic about iron and protein, but it's totally doable.

BREAKFAST

Protein smoothie (5 minutes)

Blend: 1 cup plain yogurt, 1 cup spinach, 1 cup frozen berries, 2 tbsp peanut butter, 1 tbsp chia seeds. Berries = vitamin C to help absorb iron.

LUNCH

Lentil soup + whole wheat bread (reheat)

2 cups lentil soup (made Sunday). 2 slices whole wheat bread. Side salad with pumpkin seeds.

DINNER

Tofu stir-fry (12 minutes)

Calcium-set tofu + 3 cups mixed vegetables (broccoli, peppers, bok choy) over brown rice. Top with cashews. Season with soy sauce, garlic, ginger.

What This Day Covers

Plant-based protein at every meal. Iron + vitamin C pairing. Calcium from multiple sources.

Magnesium	300+ mg	Iron	18+ mg
Zinc	9+ mg	Calcium	800+ mg
Potassium	2,500+ mg		

Sample Day #3: Minimal Cooking

For people who really, truly cannot or will not cook. Everything here can be assembled, not cooked.

BREAKFAST

Greek yogurt parfait (2 minutes)

1 cup Greek yogurt. Top with ½ cup berries and 2 tbsp pumpkin seeds. Drizzle honey if desired. No cooking. No heating.

LUNCH

Sardine salad (5 minutes)

Open can of sardines with bones. Dump on 3 cups pre-washed greens. Add rinsed chickpeas and cherry tomatoes. Top with sunflower seeds. Olive oil and vinegar. Still no cooking.

DINNER

Eggs + microwaved spinach + avocado toast (5 minutes)

Scramble 2 eggs in microwave (stir every 30 seconds for 90 seconds). Microwave 1 cup frozen spinach 2 minutes. Mash ½ avocado on 2 slices toasted whole wheat bread.

What This Day Covers

Zero actual cooking required. All minerals covered. Everything ready in minutes. Perfect for zero-energy days.

Magnesium	280+ mg	Iron	14+ mg
Zinc	10+ mg	Calcium	900+ mg
Potassium	2,400+ mg		

The Absolute Minimum Protocol (AMP)

If you're barely functioning right now, this is for you. Do only what's listed here.

Three Foods (Add These This Week)

Spinach (frozen is fine)

Microwave 1 cup for 2 minutes

Add to anything: Eggs, soup, rice, pasta

Do this 3–4 times this week

Canned black beans

Rinse them (removes sodium)

Add ½ cup to anything: Salads, rice, eggs, tacos

Do this 3–4 times this week

Pumpkin seeds

Buy a bag of roasted pumpkin seeds

Throw 2 tablespoons on anything: Yogurt, salad, oatmeal, soup

Do this daily if you can

One Supplement

Magnesium glycinate 200 mg at bedtime

That's it. Just magnesium. Take it before bed. It helps with sleep, muscle cramps, and anxiety.

If you have kidney disease or take digoxin, talk to your clinician before supplementing magnesium.

If you take warfarin (Coumadin), keep your spinach intake consistent week to week and tell your doctor about any dietary changes. Sudden increases in vitamin K affect how warfarin works.

Why Only These Things

These three foods + one supplement cover your most critical mineral needs with minimal effort:

- Spinach: Magnesium, iron, potassium
- Black beans: Iron, magnesium, zinc
- Pumpkin seeds: Magnesium, zinc
- Magnesium supplement: Fills the gap most people have

You can buy all of this at any grocery store. It's cheap. It requires almost no cooking. It takes less than 5 minutes to add these to what you're already eating.

This week: Just do these three foods and one supplement. That's your only assignment.

Don't try to do more. Just do the minimum.

The Sunday Prep Strategy (If You Have Capacity)

If you're busy during the week, spending 2 hours on Sunday will save you 10+ hours Monday through Friday.

1. Cook big batch of rice or quinoa

Put it in rice cooker or on stove. Walk away. You now have grains for the entire week.
45 minutes cooking, 5 minutes active

2. Cook big batch of beans

Use dried beans in an Instant Pot (pressure cooking mode) or boil them on the stovetop. Or just buy 3–4 cans and rinse them.

3. Prep vegetables

Wash and dry salad greens. Chop peppers, carrots, cucumbers. Store in containers.
20 minutes active

4. Hard-boil 6–12 eggs

Put eggs in water, boil 10 minutes, cool in ice water. Grab-and-go protein for the week.
15 minutes

5. Make tonight's dinner—sheet pan meal

While everything else is cooking, throw protein + potato + vegetables on a sheet pan. Tonight's dinner plus 2–3 lunches.
30 minutes cooking, 10 minutes active

What You Have Now (~60 minutes of actual work, 2 hours total)

- ✔ Grains for the week
- ✔ Beans for the week
- ✔ Prepped vegetables ready to go
- ✔ Hard-boiled eggs for quick protein
- ✔ Tonight's dinner plus leftovers

The rest of the week, you're just assembling meals using the formulas. Everything is already cooked.

Protection—Safety—Healing Check-in

You just learned about food. Before you move on, check in with yourself.

Are you overwhelmed?

Too many options? Can't process all this? You're in Protection mode—or you dropped into it during this chapter.

Here's what to do: Stop reading. Go back to the AMP above. Three foods, one supplement. That's your only job this week. The rest of this chapter will still be here when you're ready.

Are you stable?

Have some ideas about what to add this week? You're in Safety mode.

Pick one thing from this list:

- Add one of the Magnificent Seven foods you don't currently eat
- Try one meal formula once this week
- Make one batch of something on Sunday

Just one thing. Not all of it. Write it down. Do that one thing this week. Next week, add one more thing if you're ready.

Are you engaged and ready to transform your diet strategically?

You're in Healing mode. Make a plan:

- Which 2–3 Magnificent Seven foods will you add this week?
- Which meal formula will you try?
- Will you do Sunday prep?

Execute your plan. Give it 2–3 weeks. Track how you feel. Then decide if you need supplements on top of food (that's Chapter 4).

You've Finished Chapter 3

You now understand:

- ✔ Why food beats pills (and when you need both)
- ✔ The seven food categories that cover most of your mineral needs
- ✔ Simple ways to add them without elaborate cooking
- ✔ How to pace yourself based on your capacity

Your next step:

Protection mode: Do the AMP. Nothing else.

Safety mode: Add one food or try one formula this week.

Healing mode: Move to Chapter 4 to learn when supplements help and which ones matter.

You may want to bookmark this chapter or print the Magnificent Seven list and the AMP for easy reference.

You don't have to be perfect.

You don't have to do everything at once.

Adding is easier than restricting.

Progress beats perfection.

You're building your foundation.
One small change at a time. That's enough.

CHAPTER 4

Supplements: What to Buy (and What to Skip)

Supplements can help. But they're not magic pills. And they don't work for everyone, even when you're taking the right ones.

You Shouldn't Have to Guess

You've probably stood in front of a wall of bottles, completely overwhelmed. Different brands, different forms, different doses—everyone claiming their product is the best.

Maybe you've already tried supplements that didn't work. Maybe you spent money you didn't have on something that promised everything and delivered nothing. Maybe you don't know who to trust anymore.

That confusion isn't your fault. The system isn't built to make this simple.

This chapter cuts through the noise. We'll cover what actually works, what's a waste of money, and most importantly—why supplements sometimes fail even when you're taking the right ones.

Feeling overwhelmed? If this chapter starts to feel like too much, stop here and go to **Chapter 3** for the Absolute Minimum Protocol. You can come back to supplements later.

Why Supplements Don't Always Work: The Three Hidden Problems

Before we talk about what to buy, we need to talk about something most supplement books completely miss: why supplements don't always work, even when you're taking the right ones.

You can have plenty of minerals in your body and still feel terrible. Your blood tests might look fine. Your supplement bottles might be half-empty. But you're exhausted, anxious, not sleeping, still getting sick.

Here's why.

Problem #1: The Signaling Problem

Minerals don't work alone. They need signals—peptides (short chains of amino acids that act as messengers) that tell them where to go and what to do.

Think of minerals like construction workers showing up to a job site. They're ready to work. They have their tools. But if there's no foreman telling them where to go and what to build, they just stand around. The work doesn't get done, even though the workers are there.

Without adequate peptide signals, your minerals may not get where they need to go. The magnesium is in your bloodstream, but it doesn't get the message to relax your muscles or calm your nerves.

What you're looking for: Your body makes fewer of the repair and signaling peptides as you age—the ones that help your cells communicate and use nutrients properly. This decline starts in your 30s and picks up speed in your 40s, 50s, and beyond.

Problem #2: The Survival Mode Problem

When you're in chronic survival mode—Protection mode—your body literally cannot use nutrients properly.

Your body thinks a tiger is chasing you. In that moment, does your body care about building strong bones? No. Making energy for tomorrow? No. Absorbing minerals from your lunch? No.

What happens to minerals in survival mode:

- Absorption drops: Blood flow diverts away from your digestive system.
- Depletion accelerates: Stress hormones burn through magnesium, zinc, and B vitamins rapidly.
- Inflammation increases: Your body uses up minerals fighting perceived "danger."
- Signaling gets disrupted: Those peptide signals get scrambled.

The Vicious Cycle
Low minerals → Feel worse → More stress → Burn through minerals faster → Even lower levels → Feel even worse → More stress → Repeat

Problem #3: Both at Once (The Double Whammy)

Most people over 40 who are chronically stressed have BOTH problems.

- Your peptide production is declining with age (Problem #1)
- Your nervous system is stuck in survival mode (Problem #2)
- Your body is working against itself on multiple levels

What this means for your supplement strategy: Getting enough minerals is necessary but not always sufficient. You might need to address all three: minerals + signaling + nervous system.

We'll cover nervous system regulation in Chapter 5, signaling support in Chapter 6, and gut healing in Chapter 7.

When Food Isn't Enough

You already know food should come first (Chapter 3). But let's be honest about when that's not enough.

You need supplements when:

1. You're severely deficient

If your ferritin is very low, you're not eating your way out of that quickly. Same with clearly low vitamin D (under ~20 ng/mL is typically considered deficient) or magnesium. Food maintains levels. Supplements correct deficiencies.

2. You have absorption issues

Crohn's disease, celiac disease, chronic digestive issues, gastric bypass, or years on PPIs (Prilosec, Nexium). Your gut is compromised. You need higher doses in more absorbable forms.

3. You're on medications that deplete minerals

Diuretics drain potassium and magnesium. PPIs block magnesium, iron, and calcium. Metformin depletes B12. ACE inhibitors may reduce zinc levels. Food can't keep up.

4. Your needs are extreme

Pregnant women need 50% more iron—most prenatal vitamins are formulated for this, so extra supplementation is only needed if you test anemic or have low ferritin. Athletes lose minerals through sweat. Vegetarians struggle with iron absorption. Elderly people on multiple medications have everything working against them.

5. You tried food for 3 months and nothing changed

You ate beans, greens, nuts, and seeds religiously. You tracked everything. Your symptoms didn't budge. Time to supplement. Food clearly isn't enough for your situation.

The 3 Supplements Most People Actually Need

Walk into any supplement store and you'll see thousands of products. Rows and rows of bottles making promises.

You need three. Maybe four. That's it.

Quick Reference: Which Supplement Do I Need?

Supplement	Who Benefits Most	Skip If
Magnesium	Cramps, insomnia, anxiety, stress	Asymptomatic with good diet
Vitamin D	Low sun exposure, indoor workers, darker skin	Recent normal test
Iron	Heavy periods, fatigue, vegetarians	Not tested—NEVER guess

Protection mode version: If you can only do one thing, take magnesium glycinate at bedtime for 7 days. That's enough. Come back later.

Supplement #1: Magnesium

(200–400 mg daily)

Studies show roughly half of Americans don't get the RDA for magnesium from food. Soil mineral content has declined over decades. Processed foods have almost none. Stress depletes it constantly.

Get this supplement if you have: muscle cramps, insomnia, anxiety, migraines, or high blood pressure.

Best form: Magnesium glycinate. It's calming, absorbs well, and won't cause diarrhea. Don't buy the cheap magnesium oxide—it doesn't absorb well.

What you're looking for: Start with 200 mg at bedtime. If you're still having symptoms after 1 week, increase to 400 mg. Take before bed—it's calming and helps sleep.

Safety note: If you have kidney disease or take digoxin, talk to your clinician before supplementing magnesium.

Skip it if: *You reliably eat magnesium-rich foods daily and have no symptoms of deficiency.*

Supplement #2: Vitamin D

(1,000–2,000 IU daily)

Yes, this isn't technically a mineral. But it's essential for calcium absorption and mineral metabolism.

Studies estimate about 40% of Americans have insufficient vitamin D levels. For most people, food alone doesn't provide enough. Sun exposure is unreliable—sunscreen blocks it, winter exists, most people work indoors.

Get this supplement if you: work indoors, live far from the equator, have darker skin, are over 50, or use sunscreen regularly.

Best form: Vitamin D3 (cholecalciferol), not D2. D3 is what your body makes from sunlight.

What you're looking for: 1,000–2,000 IU daily for maintenance. 4,000 IU daily if you tested low (under 30 ng/mL) for 2–3 months, then retest. Take with any meal that contains fat.

Pair with K2 if supplementing calcium: If you're also taking calcium supplements, pair vitamin D3 with vitamin K2 (100–200 mcg daily). K2 helps direct calcium to bones and teeth rather than soft tissues like arteries.

⚠ **TEST FIRST. THIS IS NON-NEGOTIABLE.**

Iron is not something you guess about. Too little iron makes you exhausted. Too much iron is toxic and can damage your organs.

This isn't meant to scare you—just to keep you safe.

Supplement #3: Iron

(25–65 mg daily—ONLY if deficient)

Get tested if you have: heavy periods, chronic fatigue, hair loss, or you're vegetarian/vegan.

Best form: Ferrous bisglycinate (gentle on stomach) or carbonyl iron.

What you're looking for:

Ferritin under 20: take 65 mg

Ferritin 20–30: start with 25–50 mg

Take with: Vitamin C (orange juice or a supplement). Vitamin C dramatically increases iron absorption.

Take away from: Calcium, coffee, tea. Wait at least 2 hours. Morning with breakfast is best.

For many people, magnesium plus vitamin D covers the majority of common deficiencies. Add iron only if you tested low. Everything else is situational.

How to Choose Quality (Without Wasting Money)

Not all supplements are created equal. Some are garbage. Some are fine. Some are excellent. Here's how to tell the difference.

Look for Third-Party Testing

This is the single most important thing. These seals mean an independent lab actually tested the product:

Certification	What It Means
USP Verified	Gold standard. Rigorous testing.
NSF Certified	Widely respected. Tests for contaminants.
ConsumerLab.com	Issues CL Seal of Approved Quality; also publishes results online.
Informed-Choice	Popular for sports supplements.

No seal? Be skeptical.

Check the Form of the Mineral

Not all magnesium is magnesium. The form matters enormously.

Mineral	Good Forms	Avoid/Note
Magnesium	Glycinate, malate, threonate, taurate	Oxide (poorly absorbed; only used as a short-term laxative, not as a mineral supplement)
Iron	Ferrous bisglycinate, carbonyl iron	Ferrous sulfate (harsh)
Zinc	Picolinate, citrate, acetate, gluconate	Oxide (poorly absorbed)
Calcium	Citrate (absorbs without stomach acid)	Carbonate (needs stomach acid)

The cheap stuff uses the cheap forms. Pay a little more for forms that actually work.

Third-Party Tested Brands That Work

I'm not sponsored by any of these. These brands consistently test well:

Premium Quality: Thorne, Pure Encapsulations, Designs for Health

Solid Mid-Range: NOW Foods, Jarrow Formulas, Life Extension

Store Brands Worth Buying: Kirkland (Costco)—USP verified, Nature Made—USP verified

My Top Value Pick: NOW Foods. Good quality, third-party tested, widely available, and won't break your budget.

Any brand on this list is sufficient. There is no "perfect" choice.

What to Take, When to Take It

Timing matters. Taking things at the wrong time means they won't work as well—or at all.

Morning (with breakfast)

- Iron (if taking)—WITH orange juice, AWAY FROM calcium, coffee, tea
- B-Complex (if taking)—Energizing, not for bedtime
- Vitamin D—With a meal that contains fat

Evening (before bed)

- Magnesium—Calming, helps sleep (200–400 mg)

Critical Separations (2–4 hours apart)

Some supplements block each other's absorption. Don't take these together:

- Iron and calcium—separate by 2 hours
- Iron and coffee/tea—separate by 2 hours
- Calcium, iron, and magnesium and thyroid medication—separate by 4 hours

Sample Daily Schedule

Time	What to Take
7:00 AM	Thyroid medication (if applicable) with water ONLY
7:30 AM	Breakfast: Iron supplement + orange juice, Vitamin D
9:30 AM	Coffee (waited 2 hours after iron)
10:00 PM	Bedtime: Magnesium 200–400 mg

Essential Supplement Combinations for Specific Situations

Some situations require specific combinations. Here's what works for different needs.

For Vegetarian/Vegan

- Iron bisglycinate (25–50 mg with vitamin C)
- Zinc picolinate (15–30 mg)
- B12 sublingual (500–1,000 mcg)—non-negotiable
- Magnesium glycinate (200–400 mg)
- Vitamin D3 (1,000–2,000 IU)

Why: Plant foods don't provide adequate B12, iron absorbs poorly from plants, and zinc absorption is blocked by compounds in grains and beans.

For Over 65

- Magnesium glycinate (400 mg)
- Vitamin D3 (2,000–4,000 IU)
- Calcium citrate (500 mg, with the rest from food)
- B12 sublingual (1,000 mcg)

Why: Stomach acid decreases with age. You absorb less from food. Calcium and vitamin D protect bones. B12 prevents "dementia" symptoms that are actually deficiency.

For Pregnant

- Prenatal vitamin (specifically formulated for pregnancy)
- Extra iron if anemic (25–65 mg)
- Omega-3 DHA (for baby's brain development)

Why: You're making another human. Your needs are dramatically higher, especially iron and folate.

Budget Options: Three Tiers

Let's be realistic about cost. Here are three budget tiers that actually work.

Tier 1: Bare Minimum—$20–30/month

This covers the most common deficiencies for most people.

✔ Magnesium glycinate 200–400 mg

✔ Vitamin D3 1,000–2,000 IU

✔ Iron 25–65 mg (only if tested low)

Tier 2: Comprehensive—$40–60/month

Everything from Tier 1, plus:

✔ Zinc picolinate 15–30 mg

✔ B-complex (if vegetarian, over 50, or on metformin)

Tier 3: Optimal—$80–120/month

Everything from Tier 2, plus:

✔ Calcium citrate, under 500 mg per dose (if you don't eat dairy — see page 225 for full guidance)

✔ Vitamin K2 (pairs with D and calcium)

✔ Omega-3 fish oil (if you don't eat fatty fish 2–3x/week)

More is not better if it adds stress.

Most people do fine with Tier 1 or Tier 2. Don't go into debt buying supplements.

Feel—Pause—Act: Before You Buy Supplements

You just learned about supplements. Maybe you're already mentally adding things to your cart.

Pause.

FEEL

What's happening in your body right now? Are you feeling urgency? Pressure to "fix everything"? Rehearsing your supplement cart in your head?

PAUSE

Take a breath. Ask yourself:

- Have I actually tested to know what I'm deficient in?
- Have I tried improving my diet first for at least 4–6 weeks?
- Do I know which ONE supplement I need most?
- Am I calm enough right now to make a good decision?

If you answered NO to any of these, slow down.

ACT

Pick one action this week:

Option 1: Get tested first (Chapter 2). Know what you actually need.

Option 2: Start with magnesium + vitamin D. Safe for almost everyone.

Option 3: Add iron only if you're certain you need it.

Just one action. Not all three.

Protection—Safety—Healing Check-in

You just learned about supplements. Before you move on, check in with yourself.

Are you overwhelmed?

Too much information? Feeling stressed about this? You're in Protection mode.

Here's what to do: Stop. Close the browser. Don't order anything yet. Go to Chapter 3. Do the Absolute Minimum Protocol. Testing isn't urgent. Stabilizing is urgent.

Are you stable?

Have some clarity about what you actually need? You're in Safety mode.

Pick one action this week:

- Get tested first, then buy based on results, OR
- Buy magnesium + vitamin D and see how you feel in 8 weeks, OR
- Add iron if you're certain you need it

Just one action. Not all three.

Are you engaged and ready to be strategic?

You're in Healing mode. Make a strategic plan:

- What have you tested? What do your results show?
- Which 1–3 supplements do you actually need?
- What forms will you buy? (Check for third-party testing)
- How long will you give this before reassessing? (Minimum 8 weeks)

Execute your plan. Track your symptoms. Retest in 3 months.

You've Finished Part I

You now understand:

- ✔ Whether minerals are part of your problem (Chapter 1)
- ✔ When testing matters and how to get it (Chapter 2)
- ✔ What to eat starting now (Chapter 3)
- ✔ When supplements help and which ones matter (Chapter 4)

You have the foundation everyone needs.

Your Next Step

If you're getting tested: Schedule it, then move to Chapter 3. Don't wait for results to start eating better.

If you're skipping testing: Go directly to Chapter 3 (Food First).

Either way, Chapter 3 is next. Everyone benefits from the food foundation.

What to Remember About Supplements

- ✔ Quality matters more than quantity
- ✔ Consistency matters more than perfection
- ✔ Time matters—give it 8–12 weeks minimum
- ✔ You can't supplement your way out of a terrible diet
- ✔ Test first when possible, especially for iron
- ✔ One supplement, taken consistently, beats ten supplements taken sporadically

End of Part I: Mineral Essentials

Your Foundation Is Built

For many people, Part I is enough. If you got your ferritin and magnesium tested, started eating from the Magnificent Seven, added 1–2 targeted supplements, and did this consistently for 8–12 weeks—you might feel dramatically better.

If that's you, stop here. Keep doing what's working. Retest in 3–6 months. Come back if you get stuck or curious.

But if you're still struggling—especially if you're over 40, chronically stressed, or your tests look "fine" but you feel terrible—Part II explains why.

PART II

Understanding Your Body

When Minerals Aren't Enough

In This Section:

CHAPTER 5

Your Nervous System and Mineral Health

Why you can do everything right and still struggle—And what to do about it.

You're Not Imagining It. And You're Not Broken.

You did what they told you. Ate better. Took the supplements. Got your levels up. And you're still exhausted. Still anxious. Still not sleeping.

Nothing is wrong with you. Your body is doing what it learned to do - protecting you. The problem is, it hasn't gotten the message that the danger has passed.

This chapter explains why - and what you can do about it.

Researchers are still mapping these pathways; what follows is a practical, simplified model.

What Is Your Nervous System?

Let's start with the basics.

Your nervous system is your body's communication network. It's how your brain talks to the rest of your body, and how your body talks back to your brain.

The Physical Structure

Your brain - the control center. Your spinal cord - the main cable connecting brain to body. Billions of nerves - branching out to every part of your body: organs, muscles, skin, and glands.

These nerves carry two types of messages: messages going TO your brain (the stove is hot, my stomach is full) and messages coming FROM your brain (move your hand, start digesting that food, relax, you're safe).

What Your Nervous System Controls

Your heartbeat and breathing. Your digestion. Your immune response. Your hormones. Your body temperature. Your muscle movement. Your thoughts and emotions. Your ability to heal and repair tissue. And yes - your ability to absorb and use minerals.

Without your nervous system, nothing in your body would work.

The Two Branches: Your Gas Pedal and Brake

Your nervous system has two main branches that work together like a gas pedal and a brake.

The Gas Pedal:
Fight-or-Flight Mode

Speeds things up. Gets you ready for action.

- Increases heart rate
- Pumps blood to muscles
- Releases stress hormones
- Sharpens focus on threats
- Increases breathing rate
- Releases glucose for quick energy

The Brake:
Rest-and-Repair Mode

Slows things down. Turns on healing.

- Slows heart rate
- Decreases blood pressure
- Activates digestion
- Supports immune function
- Enables tissue repair
- Allows deep sleep
- Allows nutrient absorption

You need both systems: the gas pedal for action and emergencies, the brake for healing and restoration. Neither is inherently good or bad.

The problem happens when you get stuck with the gas pedal pressed down and the brake barely functioning.

Work stress, financial worry, relationship conflict, past trauma - all of these can keep your system in threat mode, day after day, year after year.

How This Affects Your Minerals

Let's get specific about what happens to minerals when your body is stuck in gas pedal mode.

Magnesium Gets Depleted Fast

During stress, magnesium demand rises and losses can increase - including urinary loss - which may contribute to depletion over time.

The cruel irony: Magnesium is needed to calm your nervous system. So the more stressed you are, the more magnesium you may use up, which can make you more vulnerable to stress, which depletes more magnesium.

The Vicious Cycle: Low minerals > Feel worse > More stress > Burn through minerals faster > Even lower levels > Feel even worse > Repeat

Calcium Regulation Shifts

When you're stressed, your stress hormones can decrease calcium absorption in your gut, increase calcium loss in your urine, and shift calcium regulation in ways that, over time, can contribute to bone loss. This is one reason why chronic stress is considered a risk factor for weak bones.

Other Minerals Can Suffer Too

Zinc may not work properly when you're stressed—not because it disappears, but because inflammation causes your body to move zinc out of your bloodstream and into your cells and liver. Less zinc circulating means less available to do its job. Potassium can get flushed through your kidneys. Iron availability can drop because inflammation increases hepcidin, which can reduce iron access even when total stores look adequate. Selenium gets used up fighting the oxidative stress that often comes with chronic activation.

But here's what's important: This doesn't mean minerals are useless when you're stressed. It means you may need MORE minerals while you work on nervous system regulation. The two strategies work together, not against each other.

This is why stabilization often comes before optimization - and why mineral support alone sometimes isn't enough.

The next section touches on early-life experiences. You don't need to analyze your past or excavate memories. This is simply context - not blame, not an assignment. Read what feels manageable; skip what doesn't.

The Childhood Connection

If you experienced difficult things in childhood, your nervous system may have learned that the world is generally unsafe.

There's well-known research called the Adverse Childhood Experiences Study (the ACEs Study). Researchers studied over 17,000 people and found that childhood trauma - including abuse, neglect, household dysfunction, and witnessing violence - is strongly associated with adult health outcomes decades later.

People who experienced more childhood trauma had significantly higher rates of: heart disease and diabetes, autoimmune conditions, depression and anxiety, chronic inflammation, and trouble managing stress.

The Connection to Minerals

If your nervous system learned early in life that the world isn't safe, you may have spent decades with your gas pedal pressed down. That can mean decades of stress hormones depleting minerals, poor digestion reducing mineral absorption, chronic inflammation burning through minerals faster, and disrupted sleep.

This is why some people do everything right - eat well, take supplements, exercise - and still struggle. The minerals are only part of the picture.

> **Important:** If you experienced childhood trauma, this doesn't mean you're doomed. It means you have an extra layer to work with. And your nervous system can absolutely heal and change, even after decades. Your brain and nervous system can form new patterns. It takes intentional work, but it's possible.

What Safety Actually Means

When most people think about creating safety for their nervous system, they think about reducing external stress, doing breathing exercises, creating a calm environment, or avoiding anything upsetting.

Those things can help. But they're not what safety actually means.

> **Real safety for your nervous system means: having the capacity to feel whatever emotions arise - fear, anger, sadness, shame, joy, grief - without judging yourself, pushing them away, or being overwhelmed by them.**

This is completely different from trying to feel calm all the time or avoiding anything that might upset you.

Think about it: When you were a child and something scary or upsetting happened, were you allowed to feel those feelings? Or did you learn that big emotions weren't allowed, that crying was weakness, that anger was dangerous, that fear meant you were too sensitive?

Most of us learned that certain emotions weren't safe to feel. So we developed ways to avoid them: stay busy, numb out with food or scrolling, disconnect from your body, push through and ignore what you're feeling, judge yourself harshly.

Here's the problem: When you can't safely feel your emotions, your nervous system stays in survival mode. The unfelt emotions don't go away. They get stored in your body as chronic muscle tension, digestive problems, pain, inflammation, stress hormones that won't turn off, sleep problems - and yes, mineral depletion and poor mineral absorption.

Real nervous system regulation isn't about feeling calm all the time. It's about being able to feel whatever is actually happening inside you.

Feel—Pause—Act: How Nervous System Regulation Works

Feel-Pause-Act draws on a wide body of research in nervous system regulation. Studies consistently show that accepting difficult emotions—rather than avoiding them—tends to reduce distress, while suppression keeps the nervous system stuck.

That's exactly what Feel-Pause-Act teaches you to do.

Feel: Creating Safety to Actually Feel

The first step is practicing feeling whatever is happening in your body right now. Not analyzing it. Not fixing it. Not making it go away. Just feeling it.

Most people are disconnected from their body's signals. They've learned to override discomfort, push through fatigue, ignore warning signs.

Feel asks you to: Notice what sensations are present in your body right now. Acknowledge whatever emotion is there without judgment. Stay present with it for even just a few breaths.

Signs of Gas Pedal Mode

- Shallow, fast breathing
- Tight jaw or shoulders
- Clenched fists or tense muscles
- Racing thoughts
- Can't sit still
- Heart pounding
- Stomach upset
- Feeling wired or on edge

Signs of Brake Mode

- Slow, deep breathing
- Relaxed muscles
- Calm, clear thoughts
- Can be still comfortably
- Steady heartbeat
- Comfortable digestion
- Feeling grounded or at ease

The key: Whatever you notice is okay. You're not trying to change from one state to another. You're just noticing. The simple act of feeling - of being present with your actual experience without judgment - begins to create safety in your nervous system.

Pause: Creating Space Between Feeling and Reacting

The second step is creating a gap between what you feel and how you respond. This is where choice enters.

When you're stuck in survival mode, there's no gap. Something triggers you, and you immediately react: snap at someone, shut down and withdraw, reach for food or your phone to numb out, push through and ignore what you're feeling, spiral into anxiety.

The pause interrupts that automatic pattern.

After you've noticed what you're feeling (the Feel step), you pause. You don't act on it immediately. You don't push it down. You just create space.

This pause might be: Three deep breaths. Placing your hand on your heart or belly. Counting to ten. Stepping outside for a moment. Simply sitting with the sensation for 60–90 seconds.

During this pause, you're not trying to talk yourself out of the feeling or think your way through it. You're just being with it. Letting it exist. Giving it space.

Many emotions rise and fall faster than we expect when we stop resisting them - sometimes within a minute or two. The exact timing varies, but the principle is consistent: allowing the wave helps it move.

Most people never discover this because they either push the emotion down or get swept away by it before it can pass. The pause lets you stay present long enough for the nervous system to complete its cycle.

Act: Choosing Your Response

The third step is choosing what to do next based on awareness rather than automatic pattern.

After you've felt what's present and paused to create space, you choose your response. This might be: A practice that helps (breath work, movement, going outside). Having a difficult conversation you've been avoiding. Setting a boundary. Asking for help. Doing nothing - just continuing to be with the feeling. Taking action that aligns with your values rather than your fear.

The key difference: You're acting from awareness rather than reacting from survival mode.

You're not pushing the feeling down (which keeps you stuck). You're not being controlled by the feeling (which leads to overwhelm or impulsive reactions). You're making a conscious choice about what serves you in this moment.

Example: Feel-Pause-Act in Real Life

Without Feel-Pause-Act

You're reading about how chronic stress depletes magnesium and realize you've been in fight-or-flight mode for years.

Immediately, you feel a wave of shame and hopelessness.

I've ruined my health. It's too late.

You close the book, order takeout, and tell yourself you'll deal with it later.

With Feel-Pause-Act

You're reading about chronic stress and feel that same wave of shame rise (Feel).

You notice your chest tightening, tears starting. Instead of closing the book, you pause.

You put your hand on your chest and take three slow breaths. You let yourself feel the grief without judging it (Pause).

Then you choose: maybe you call someone who helps you feel grounded, or you go for a walk (Act).

The grief might still be there. But you're not running from it or drowning in it. You're acknowledging what's true AND taking steps to heal. That's regulation. That's how change happens.

When You Need Extra Support

Sometimes you're too activated to simply Feel-Pause-Act. Your survival mode is running too high, or you're so shut down you can't feel anything.

That's where support practices come in. These aren't regulation themselves. They're tools that help you access Feel-Pause-Act when you're too dysregulated to do it on your own.

For High Activation (gas pedal floored)

Breath work: Slow, deep breathing activates your brake system. Try breathing in for 4 counts, out for 6 counts, for a few minutes. The longer exhale tells your body it's safe to slow down.

Cold water: Splash cold water on your face or hold ice on your neck. This immediately activates your brake system. It's a fast reset. (If you have cardiovascular concerns, use gentler temperature shifts and check with your clinician.)

Movement: Sometimes you need to move the activation through your body first. Shaking, a brisk walk, or jumping jacks can discharge excess energy so you can then Feel-Pause-Act.

For Numbness or Shutdown

Grounding: Use your five senses to come back into your body. Name 5 things you can see, 4 you can touch, 3 you can hear, 2 you can smell, 1 you can taste.

Gentle movement: Sometimes gentle stretching or a slow walk helps you reconnect with your body when you're numb or disconnected.

Ongoing Supports

Safe relationships: Your nervous system regulates in relationship with other calm, safe people. Spending time with people who feel safe helps your system settle.

Time in nature: Research suggests that even 20 minutes in nature can help reduce stress hormones.

Quality sleep: When you're well-rested, everything becomes easier.

Professional support: Sometimes, especially with significant trauma history, you need professional help. Approaches like Somatic Experiencing, EMDR, Internal Family Systems, or trauma-informed therapy can be life-changing.

Why This Matters for Minerals

Your body absorbs and uses minerals better when it feels safe.

And by safe, I mean enough internal capacity to feel what you feel without overwhelm.

This doesn't mean you have to be perfectly regulated before minerals work. They still help even when you're stressed. But they work BETTER - sometimes dramatically better - when your nervous system isn't constantly in survival mode.

When your body feels safe:

Digestion works properly | Nutrients are absorbed efficiently | Hormones balance | Immune function works | Tissue repair happens | Minerals can do their jobs

There's another layer: signaling. Minerals don't just show up - your body has to direct them. That's Chapter 6.

Nervous system regulation and mineral supplementation are partners, not competitors. Do both. They amplify each other.

Protection—Safety—Healing Check-in

You just learned about your nervous system. Before you move on, notice where you are.

Feeling overwhelmed? This was a lot of information?

That's okay. You don't need to master Feel-Pause-Act today. Just notice it exists. Try it once this week - just once. Notice what you're feeling right now. Pause. That's enough.

Feeling stable? Some of this resonated?

Good. You understand how your nervous system affects mineral health. Try practicing Feel-Pause-Act a few times this week. Just notice, pause, choose. See what happens.

Feeling engaged? Ready to go deeper?

Excellent. You understand the pattern - and how to work with it. Practice Feel-Pause-Act daily. Consider whether professional support might help you go further. Keep reading - the next chapters build on this foundation.

What You Need to Remember

Your nervous system influences whether your body can absorb and use minerals effectively.

It has two modes: fight-or-flight (gas pedal) and rest-and-repair (brake). When you're stuck in fight-or-flight, minerals can get depleted faster and may not work as well.

Real safety for your nervous system means the capacity to feel emotions without judgment, suppression, or overwhelm.

Feel-Pause-Act is how nervous system regulation actually works: Feel what's present, Pause before reacting, Act from awareness.

Other practices (breath work, cold water, movement) are supports that help you access Feel-Pause-Act when you're too dysregulated.

Minerals still help even when your nervous system isn't perfectly regulated - but they tend to work better when you're not in constant survival mode.

CHAPTER 6

The Missing Signal

Why minerals don't always work—even when you're doing everything right.

This Isn't Your Fault

You followed the advice. Took the supplements. Changed your diet. Got your levels checked. And you're still not feeling better.

You might be wondering if you're doing something wrong. If you're somehow broken. If everyone else gets results except you.

You're not broken. And you're not doing it wrong. There's a piece of the puzzle that most people - including most doctors - don't know about.

This chapter explains what it is.

The Mineral Paradox: Normal Levels, Terrible Symptoms

You've been taking magnesium for months. Your blood tests show normal levels. But you're still exhausted, still having muscle cramps, still struggling with sleep.

What's going on?

Here's what most doctors won't tell you: having enough minerals in your body doesn't mean your body knows what to do with them.

Think of it this way: You can have a fully stocked toolbox in your garage, but if no one tells the tools what to build, they just sit there. Your minerals are the same way. They need instructions. They need signals telling them where to go, what to do, and when to do it.

Researchers have documented something puzzling for years: people with normal mineral levels on blood tests who still experience all the symptoms of deficiency.

Some people with normal mineral levels on blood tests still experience symptoms of deficiency. This isn't rare. It points to a signaling problem—the minerals are present but aren't being directed efficiently to where they're needed.

This isn't rare. It's common.

Here's what was happening: their bodies had the minerals. They just didn't have enough signals telling those minerals what to do.

This is the mineral paradox. You can have adequate mineral levels and still experience symptoms. Not because you don't have enough minerals, but because your body's signaling system isn't working optimally.

The missing piece is signaling. Peptides are one of the most overlooked parts of that signal.

What Are Peptides?

Let's break this down simply.

Your body is constantly sending messages. Build muscle here. Repair this tissue. Use this mineral for energy production. Send calcium to build bone.

Many of those messages are carried by peptides—one of the body's key signaling tools.

The Building Blocks

Peptides are short chains of amino acids — fewer than about 50 of them. Proteins are longer chains, generally 50 amino acids or more. Both are built from the same amino acid building blocks, but they're different molecules with different jobs.

Think of it like this: Amino acids are individual letters. Peptides are words. Proteins are sentences. Related, but not the same thing.

Peptides carry specific, important messages.

Your body makes thousands of different peptides, and each one carries a specific instruction. Some tell your cells to grow. Some tell your immune system to calm down. Some tell your body to heal damaged tissue.

And many of them help direct how minerals are used in your body.

Why Haven't You Heard About Them?

Because until recently, we didn't have great ways to study them. They're tiny. They break down quickly. They're hard to measure. So while researchers knew peptides existed, they were mostly a mystery.

That's changing now. We're learning that peptides are one of the most important signaling systems in your body.

How Signals Tell Minerals What to Do

Minerals don't just float around in your body waiting to be helpful. They need to be directed to specific places, activated in specific ways, and told when to work.

That's part of what peptides do.

Example: Magnesium and Muscle Function

You have magnesium in your bloodstream. Your muscle cells need that magnesium to relax properly after contracting. But the magnesium doesn't just know to go into your muscle cells.

A peptide signals your muscle cells to open their doors and let the magnesium in. Another peptide activates the enzymes that use magnesium for energy production. Without those signals, the magnesium circulates but doesn't do its job as efficiently.

Example: Iron and Energy Production

Iron carries oxygen to your cells for energy production. But getting iron into the right places requires a peptide called hepcidin that regulates how much iron gets absorbed from food and released from storage. If peptide signaling is suboptimal, you might have adequate iron stores but not use them as efficiently.

> **See the pattern? Minerals are the raw materials. Signals tell your body how to use them. Peptides are one of those signals. You need both.**

The Age Factor: Why Signaling Declines

Here's the part that really matters: your body naturally produces fewer peptides as you age.

It's not your fault. It's biology.

What Contributes to This Decline

Your body produces less growth hormone (which stimulates production of other peptides). Cellular energy production slows. Accumulated inflammation interferes with signaling pathways. Chronic stress suppresses peptide production.

In Your 30s

Peptide production starts to slow down. Most people don't notice yet because the decline is gradual and your body compensates well. You might notice recovery from workouts takes a little longer, or stress affects you more than it did in your 20s.

In Your 40s

The decline accelerates. This is when many people start experiencing symptoms they can't explain: persistent fatigue despite normal lab results, loss of muscle mass even with exercise, slower metabolism, brain fog, poor recovery from exercise or illness. This is often when the mineral paradox shows up. You supplement with minerals, your levels look fine, but you don't feel as good as expected.

In Your 50s and Beyond

Peptide decline continues. Many people are told their symptoms are just aging. But often, what they're experiencing is the compound effect of both mineral status AND peptide signaling changes. Sleep quality often declines (many peptides are produced during deep sleep).

An Important Clarification

I want to be clear about something: declining peptide signaling doesn't mean minerals stop working.

It means they might work LESS EFFICIENTLY than they did when you were younger. It means you might need to do more to get the same results. It means addressing signaling can help you get MORE benefit from the minerals you're taking.

But minerals still help. Always.

If your signaling is suboptimal and you're ALSO mineral deficient, you'll feel worse than if your signaling is suboptimal but your mineral levels are good. Replenishing minerals is still the right first step.

Think of it like this: If your construction crew (peptides) is understaffed, they'll still build more with adequate materials (minerals) than with no materials at all. The building might go up slower. But it WILL go up.

Signs Your Signaling System Might Need Support

How do you know if peptide signaling might be part of your picture?

Look for this pattern: You're doing the basics well but not getting the results you expected.

Physical Signs

- You supplement with minerals but still have some symptoms
- Lab work shows normal levels but you don't feel great
- Exercise doesn't build muscle like it used to
- Recovery takes longer than expected
- Minor injuries heal slowly

Mental Signs

- Brain fog that persists
- Memory issues (losing train of thought, forgetting names)
- Difficulty concentrating
- Mental fatigue even when well-rested

Metabolic Signs

- Blood sugar issues despite eating well
- Difficulty losing weight even with consistent effort
- Loss of muscle mass despite resistance training

If you're nodding at several items on this list AND you're over 40, signaling support might help you get more from your mineral strategy.

What You Can Do About It

Good news: You're not powerless here.

While peptide production naturally declines with age, you can support your body's ability to make and use peptides more effectively.

Support Through Food

Your body makes peptides from amino acids (the building blocks of protein). If you're not getting enough high-quality protein, you can't make adequate peptides.

How much protein? More than most people eat, especially over 40. A reasonable target: about 0.7 to 1 gram of protein per pound of ideal body weight. If your ideal weight is 150 pounds, that's roughly 105–150 grams of protein daily.

Best sources: grass-fed beef, wild-caught fish (especially salmon, sardines), pastured eggs, organic poultry, bone broth or collagen.

For vegetarians: combine plant proteins carefully to get complete amino acid profiles.

Resistance Training

This is huge. Resistance training (weights, bodyweight exercises, resistance bands) is one of the most powerful ways to stimulate peptide production.

When you challenge your muscles with resistance, your body responds by increasing production of peptides that support growth, repair, and rebuilding.

You don't need to become a bodybuilder. But you do need to consistently challenge your muscles beyond what they're used to: 2–3 sessions per week, focus on compound movements (squats, rows, presses), gradually increase difficulty over time.

Sleep: When Peptides Are Made

Many critical peptides - including growth-supporting peptides and tissue repair peptides - are produced during deep sleep.

If your sleep is poor, your peptide production suffers.

What helps: Consistent sleep schedule. Dark, cool room. No screens for 1–2 hours before bed. Magnesium before bed (supports both sleep AND peptide production). Managing stress.

Strategic Fasting

Intermittent fasting can support certain types of peptide production. When you fast for 16+ hours, your body shifts into repair mode and increases production of peptides that support cellular cleanup and regeneration.

Practical approach: Stop eating 2–3 hours before bed. Don't eat breakfast immediately in the morning. Aim for a 12–16 hour overnight fast.

> **Important caution:** Fasting isn't appropriate for everyone. If you have a history of eating disorders, blood sugar issues, or severe stress, fasting might make things worse. Listen to your body.

When Natural Support Isn't Enough

Sometimes optimizing diet, exercise, and sleep isn't enough.

If you've made these changes and you're still struggling, it might be time to work with a practitioner who understands peptide support.

Most conventional doctors weren't trained in therapeutic peptide support—it falls outside standard clinical practice. You'll likely need to work with a functional or integrative medicine practitioner.

There are many types of peptides being used in clinical practice. Some are well-studied with decades of research. Others are newer. The field is evolving rapidly.

If you're interested in exploring peptide support, work with a knowledgeable practitioner who can help you understand current options, what the research shows, and what might be appropriate for your specific situation.

Why This Matters for Everything Else

Here's why understanding peptides matters for your mineral health:

You get MORE benefit from minerals when your signaling is working well.

All the strategies in this book - eating mineral-rich foods, supplementing wisely, addressing gut health, managing stress - work better when your peptide signaling is functioning well.

But they still work even when signaling isn't perfect. You're not wasting your time with minerals if you haven't optimized peptides. You're building the foundation that makes everything else possible.

The Three Partners:

- Minerals are the construction materials
- Peptides are the crew giving instructions
- Nervous system regulation (Chapter 5) creates the safe environment where construction can happen

You need all three for optimal results. But having ANY of them is better than having none.

Protection—Safety—Healing Check-in

You just learned about peptides and signaling. Before you move on, notice where you are.

Feeling overwhelmed? Too much science?

That's okay. Here's what matters: if you're over 40 and minerals aren't working as well as expected, signaling might be part of the picture. Eat more protein. Lift some weights. Sleep better. That's the simple version.

Feeling stable? This explains some things?

Good. You understand why minerals sometimes work better for some people than others. Focus on the lifestyle basics - protein, resistance training, sleep. These support peptide production naturally.

Feeling engaged? Want to optimize?

Excellent. Consider tracking your protein intake to ensure you're hitting 0.7–1g per pound of ideal body weight. Start or intensify resistance training. Prioritize sleep quality. If lifestyle changes aren't enough, explore working with a knowledgeable practitioner.

What You Need to Remember

Your body needs both raw materials (minerals) and instructions (peptides) to function optimally.

Peptides are short chains of amino acids that carry messages telling minerals where to go and what to do.

As you age, peptide production naturally declines, which can make minerals less efficient - but minerals still help significantly.

You can support peptide production through adequate protein intake, resistance training, quality sleep, and strategic fasting.

The strategies throughout this book work even when signaling isn't perfect - but they work BETTER when signaling is supported.

CHAPTER 7

Your Gut: The Gateway for Minerals

Why what you eat might not be reaching your bloodstream—and how to fix it.

One More Thing to Fix?

You're eating mineral-rich foods. You're taking quality supplements. Maybe you've even started working on nervous system regulation. And you're still not seeing the results you expected.

It's frustrating. And it might feel like there's always one more thing standing between you and feeling better.

But here's the truth: your gut might be the reason nothing else has worked yet. Not because you're broken - but because everything you've been putting into your body hasn't been getting through.

This chapter explains the gateway - and how to open it.

What Is Your Gut?

Your gut is your entire digestive tract - the tube that runs from your mouth to your colon.

Your Stomach

Where food gets broken down by acid and enzymes. This is especially important for mineral absorption because stomach acid helps release minerals from food.

Your Small Intestine

Where most nutrient absorption happens. This is about 20 feet long and lined with millions of tiny finger-like projections called villi (pronounced VIL-eye) that grab nutrients and pull them into your bloodstream.

Your Large Intestine (Colon)

Where water is absorbed and waste is formed. This is also where trillions of bacteria live that help with final stages of digestion.

The Gut Lining

A single layer of cells that separates the inside of your digestive tract from your bloodstream. This barrier decides what gets absorbed and what stays out.

When Your Gut Is Healthy

- Produces enough stomach acid to break down food and release minerals
- Has healthy villi to absorb nutrients efficiently
- Maintains a strong gut lining that lets nutrients through but keeps harmful things out
- Hosts beneficial bacteria that support digestion and mineral absorption

When Your Gut Is Damaged

- Low stomach acid leaves minerals trapped in food
- Damaged villi reduce absorption surface area
- Leaky gut lining lets harmful things through while damaged villi reduce nutrient absorption
- Imbalanced bacteria impair digestion

How Your Gut Absorbs Minerals

Step 1: Breaking Down Food

Your stomach produces hydrochloric acid that kills harmful bacteria in food, breaks down protein, and - critically - releases minerals from food so they can be absorbed.

Here's the problem: Many people (especially as they age) don't produce enough stomach acid. Low stomach acid means minerals stay bound up in food and can't be absorbed as well.

Common signs of low stomach acid: Feeling full or bloated after eating. Heartburn or acid reflux (counter intuitively, this can sometimes be LOW acid, not high—particularly in older adults and long-term PPI users). Undigested food in your stool. Burping or gas shortly after meals.

Step 2: Absorption in the Small Intestine

After your stomach, partially digested food moves to your small intestine. This is where most mineral absorption happens.

Your small intestine is lined with millions of villi - tiny finger-like projections that dramatically increase surface area for absorption. Think of them like the fibers on a towel that soak up water.

Many things can damage these villi, making them flat, inflamed, or less efficient. When villi are damaged, absorption drops.

Research shows that people with damaged gut linings can absorb significantly less of the minerals they consume, even from supplements.

Step 3: The Gut Lining Barrier

Your gut lining is only one cell thick. It's supposed to let nutrients through while keeping out bacteria, toxins, and undigested food particles.

When the gut lining is healthy, it has tight junctions between cells that control what passes through.

When the gut lining is damaged (what researchers call increased intestinal permeability - meaning the barrier has become more porous than it should be), those tight junctions become loose. Now things that shouldn't get through can enter your bloodstream.

This triggers inflammation, which further impairs mineral absorption and increases mineral depletion.

What Damages Your Gut

Many things. And often it's a combination of factors over time.

Chronic Stress

Remember Chapter 5 on the nervous system? When you're stuck in fight-or-flight mode, your body diverts blood away from your digestive system.

Chronic stress: Reduces stomach acid production. Slows gut motility (movement of food through your system). Damages the gut lining. Changes the balance of gut bacteria. Increases inflammation.

This is why nervous system regulation (Chapter 5) comes first. If your nervous system is stuck in survival mode, your gut can't heal as well.

Medications

Proton pump inhibitors (PPIs): Drugs like omeprazole (Prilosec), esomeprazole (Nexium), and lansoprazole (Prevacid) that reduce stomach acid. They dramatically reduce the acid needed to release minerals from food. Long-term PPI use is associated with magnesium, calcium, iron, and B12 issues.

NSAIDs: Pain relievers like ibuprofen and naproxen. These can damage the gut lining and cause bleeding that depletes iron.

Antibiotics: While sometimes necessary, antibiotics kill both harmful and beneficial gut bacteria. Repeated antibiotic use disrupts gut bacterial balance for months or years.

Important: If you're on any of these long-term, talk with your doctor about whether they're still necessary and what you can do to protect your gut health.

Foods That Can Damage the Gut

Gluten: For people with celiac disease or non-celiac gluten sensitivity, gluten damages the villi in the small intestine. Even without celiac disease, some people react to gluten with inflammation.

Processed foods and sugar: High intake of processed foods, refined sugar, and industrial seed oils promotes inflammation and can damage the gut lining.

Alcohol: Regular or excessive alcohol consumption damages the gut lining, reduces stomach acid production, and depletes minerals (especially magnesium, zinc, and B vitamins).

Infections

Gut infections - bacterial, parasitic, fungal, or viral - can damage the gut lining and impair absorption.

SIBO (small intestinal bacterial overgrowth): When bacteria that normally live in the colon overgrow in the small intestine. Causes gas, bloating, and absorption issues.

H. pylori: A bacteria that infects the stomach, reduces stomach acid production, and impairs mineral absorption.

If you have persistent digestive symptoms despite dietary changes, it's worth working with a practitioner to test for infections.

Signs Your Gut Is Affecting Mineral Absorption

Look for these patterns:

Digestive Symptoms

- Bloating, gas, or discomfort after eating
- Heartburn or acid reflux
- Constipation or diarrhea (or alternating)
- Undigested food in stool
- Feeling full quickly

Mineral Symptoms Despite Supplementation

- You're taking minerals but levels stay low
- You're eating mineral-rich foods but still have deficiency symptoms
- Your response to supplements is inconsistent

History Signs to Watch For:

- History of prolonged antibiotic use
- History of gut infections
- Long-term use of PPIs or NSAIDs
- High stress lifestyle

If you're nodding at several of these, gut healing needs to be part of your strategy.

How to Heal Your Gut

Good news: Your gut can heal. The gut lining replaces itself every few days. With the right support, damaged villi can regenerate. Gut bacteria balance can be restored.

It takes time, but it's possible.

Here's a framework that works:

1. REMOVE: Take Out What's Damaging

You can't heal your gut while continuing to damage it.

Address Chronic Stress: Practice Feel-Pause-Act (Chapter 5). When you're chronically stressed, everything you do to heal your gut will be less effective.

Review Medications: Talk with your doctor about whether you still need PPIs, alternatives to regular NSAID use, and protecting your gut if you need antibiotics.

Identify Problem Foods: Consider eliminating common gut irritants for 3–4 weeks to see if symptoms improve: Gluten, Dairy (if lactose intolerant), Processed foods and refined sugar, Alcohol, Any foods you suspect trigger symptoms. After 3–4 weeks, you can systematically reintroduce foods one at a time to see what you tolerate.

Address Infections: If you suspect gut infections (persistent symptoms despite dietary changes), work with a practitioner to test and treat appropriately.

2. REPAIR: Support Gut Lining Healing

Once you've removed major irritants, support your gut's natural healing process.

Healing Foods:

- Bone broth: Rich in collagen, gelatin, and amino acids that support gut lining repair. Drink 1–2 cups daily.
- Fermented foods: Sauerkraut, kimchi, kefir, yogurt contain beneficial bacteria. Start small if you're not used to them.
- Cooked vegetables: Easier to digest than raw. Focus on well-cooked carrots, squash, zucchini, and leafy greens.
- Healthy fats: Omega-3 fats from wild fish and fish oil reduce gut inflammation.

Targeted Supplements (if gut damage is significant):

- L-glutamine: An amino acid that's the primary fuel for gut lining cells. Typical dose: 5–10 grams daily. Talk to your doctor first if you have liver disease, a history of cancer, or seizure disorders—glutamine isn't right for everyone.
- Zinc carnosine: A specific form of zinc that supports gut lining healing. Typical dose: 75–150 mg daily.
- Collagen or gelatin: Provides amino acids that support gut lining structure. Typical dose: 10–20 grams daily.
- Digestive enzymes: If you have signs of low stomach acid or poor digestion, these can help break down food while your gut heals.

3. RESTORE: Rebuild Healthy Gut Bacteria

Supporting beneficial bacteria helps with digestion, mineral absorption, and maintaining gut lining health.

Prebiotic Foods (feed beneficial bacteria): Garlic and onions, Asparagus, Slightly green bananas, Cooked and cooled potatoes or rice.

Probiotic Foods (provide beneficial bacteria): Sauerkraut, Kimchi, Kefir (if dairy tolerated), Kombucha (in moderation), Naturally fermented pickles.

Probiotic Supplements: High-quality probiotics can help restore bacterial balance, especially after antibiotics. Look for multi-strain formulas with at least 10–50 billion CFUs. Take consistently for at least 2–3 months.

Lifestyle Support: Adequate sleep (poor sleep disrupts gut bacteria), Regular moderate movement (supports gut motility), Time in nature (exposes you to diverse bacteria), Reduce unnecessary antibacterial products.

How Long Does Gut Healing Take?

This varies depending on how damaged your gut is and what caused the damage.

Mild Damage

4–8 weeks
(mainly from stress and poor diet): 4–8 weeks of focused gut healing can make a significant difference.

Moderate Damage

3–6 months
(from long-term medication use, infections, or food sensitivities): 3–6 months of consistent support.

Severe Damage

6–12 months or longer
(from untreated celiac disease, chronic infections, or decades of gut-damaging factors): 6–12 months or longer.

The key is consistency. And remember: you're not just healing your gut. You're simultaneously working on nervous system regulation and replenishing minerals. All of these support each other.

Why Gut Health Is Foundational

You can't absorb what your gut can't process.

You could eat all the mineral-rich foods in the world. You could take the highest quality supplements. But if your gut can't produce enough stomach acid, maintain healthy villi, keep the gut lining intact, and support beneficial bacteria - then those minerals won't get where they need to go as efficiently.

Heal your gut, and everything else becomes easier.

Protection—Safety—Healing Check-in

You just learned about gut health. Before you move on, notice where you are.

Feeling overwhelmed? Gut healing sounds like a lot?

That's okay. Start with just ONE thing: add bone broth or fermented foods. Don't try to implement everything. One change at a time.

Feeling stable? Have some gut issues to address?

Good. You understand the framework. Start with Remove - identify what's damaging your gut. Then add Repair foods. Then work on Restore. Give it 4–8 weeks before expecting significant changes.

Feeling engaged? Ready for comprehensive gut healing?

Excellent. Consider working with a functional medicine practitioner to test for infections or SIBO if you have persistent symptoms. Implement the full Remove-Repair-Restore framework. Track your progress over 3–6 months.

What You Need to Remember

Your gut is the gateway for mineral absorption. It includes your stomach (where acid releases minerals from food), your small intestine (where absorption happens through villi), and your gut lining (which controls what enters your bloodstream).

Many things damage gut health: chronic stress, medications like PPIs and NSAIDs, inflammatory foods, infections, and poor gut bacteria balance.

Gut healing follows a Remove-Repair-Restore framework: remove what's damaging, repair the gut lining with healing foods and targeted support, and restore healthy gut bacteria.

Gut healing takes time (weeks to months depending on severity) but is foundational for mineral absorption.

PART III

When Symptoms Speak

What Your Body Is Telling You

CHAPTER 8

Pain, Cramps, and Muscle Function

When your body won't let you rest

Two in the morning. You jolt awake with a calf cramp so painful you're gasping. Your muscle is rock-hard, twisted into a knot. You hobble around trying to stretch it out, swearing under your breath.

Or maybe it's your legs at night. They won't stay still. That creepy-crawly restless feeling deep inside drives you insane. You can't get comfortable. Can't sleep.

So you talked to your doctor. They told you: "Drink more water." "Stretch before bed." "It happens as you get older." "Try magnesium" (but didn't say how much or what kind). "Everyone gets cramps sometimes."

You left feeling dismissed.

Here's what nobody told you: Your muscles are electrochemical machines. They need precise amounts of calcium, magnesium, potassium, and iron to contract, relax, and recover properly. Mess up this balance, and your muscles start screaming—through cramps, through pain, through that maddening restless legs feeling that won't let you sleep.

Standard blood work doesn't catch this. Doctors aren't trained to look for it. So you suffer while the real problem goes untreated.

This chapter will show you what's actually happening, why it was missed, and how to work with your doctor to address it.

They Said It Was Just Aging—They Were Wrong

"Everyone gets leg cramps as they age."

TRUTH: Nighttime cramps aren't normal aging. They're usually magnesium deficiency. Magnesium is required for muscle relaxation—it's literally the off switch. When you're low, muscles can't fully release.

Replenishing it helps many people. Not stretching. Not drinking more water. Magnesium. That said, how much it helps depends on whether deficiency is your actual issue. Not stretching. Not drinking more water. Magnesium.

"Restless legs are common, especially in women."

TRUTH: Restless legs aren't "just something that happens." They're usually low iron. Studies show that when people with Restless Legs Syndrome bring their ferritin (stored iron) above 75, symptoms improve significantly—sometimes completely resolve. But doctors rarely check ferritin for restless legs. They prescribe medications instead.

"You just need to stretch more."

TRUTH: Chronic muscle tension isn't just stress. It's often a calcium-magnesium imbalance. When you don't have enough magnesium to balance calcium, your muscles contract but can't fully relax. You walk around in a state of permanent tension.

Why it gets dismissed: Doctors are trained to look for serious disease—ALS, MS, neuropathy. When those tests come back normal, they assume you're fine. What they're not trained to look for: basic mineral deficiencies that cause significant symptoms but don't qualify as medical emergencies.

You were right to seek help. Your symptoms are real. The problem isn't you.

The Muscle Switch

Here's the concept that explains everything in this chapter. Think of your muscles like a light switch with three settings:

CALCIUM	MAGNESIUM	POTASSIUM
=	=	=
ON	**OFF**	**REGULATOR**
Makes muscles contract.	Makes muscles relax.	Keeps the on/off switch
Tightens everything up.	Releases the squeeze.	working correctly.
Says "WORK!"	**Says "REST!"**	**Prevents misfires.**

You need all three. Not just one.

When the Muscle Switch Breaks Down

Too much calcium without enough magnesium?

Your switch is stuck ON. Muscles contract but can't release. Result: cramps, spasms, permanent tension, that tight knotted feeling that won't let go.

Not enough potassium?

The switch misfires. Electrical signals get scrambled. Result: random twitching, cramps out of nowhere, muscles firing when they shouldn't.

Low iron?

Your muscles don't get enough oxygen. They fatigue fast. Recover slowly. And in the case of restless legs, the wiring that controls movement signals goes haywire.

Remember The Muscle Switch. It explains why you cramp at 2 AM (switch stuck ON). It explains why your shoulders are always tight (same thing). It explains restless legs (faulty wiring from low iron). Every muscle problem in this chapter comes back to this switch.

Why Cramps Are a Warning Sign

Most people think cramps are just annoying. A minor inconvenience.

But cramps are your body's warning system. They're telling you something important: your mineral balance is off. And if it's off enough to cause cramps, other things are probably going wrong too.

What Else Might Be Happening

- Your cardiovascular system is stressed. Potassium and magnesium regulate heart rhythm. Low levels increase risk of arrhythmias.
- Your sleep quality is suffering. Even without cramps waking you, low magnesium disrupts deep sleep.
- Your stress response is dysregulated. Magnesium helps regulate stress hormones. When it's low, you stay in fight-or-flight mode.

The bottom line: Don't dismiss cramps as "just one of those things." They're information. Fix the cramps, and you'll probably fix a lot of other things you didn't even realize were problems.

Restless Legs Syndrome: When the Wiring Goes Wrong

If you have restless legs, pay very close attention to this section. What I'm about to tell you could end years of suffering.

You lie down to sleep. Within minutes, your legs start feeling weird. Not painful exactly—more like a creepy-crawly sensation deep inside. An overwhelming urge to move them. You try to stay still. You can't. You get up and walk around. The feeling goes away. You lie back down. Within minutes, it's back.

You can't sleep. You're exhausted but your legs won't let you rest.

What's Happening

Remember The Muscle Switch? Restless legs isn't about the switch itself—it's about the wiring that controls it.

Your brain needs iron to make dopamine. Dopamine controls movement and the perception of movement in your legs. When iron is low—even "low normal"—dopamine production drops. Movement signals get scrambled. Result: your legs feel weird, won't stay still, and you can't sleep.

THE NUMBER YOUR DOCTOR DOESN'T KNOW

If you have restless legs, remember this number:

Ferritin above 75

Not above 15 (where "normal" starts on lab ranges). Not above 30. **Above 75.**

Write this number down. Take it to your appointment.

Research consistently shows RLS symptoms improve—sometimes completely resolve—when ferritin reaches this threshold. But most doctors see ferritin of 20 or 25 and say "your iron is fine."

It's not fine. Not for this.

The Magnesium Piece

Many people with RLS also have low magnesium. The Muscle Switch is involved too—magnesium helps with the "can't relax" component, the tension and inability to calm down.

Some people find that fixing iron alone solves it. Others need both iron and magnesium. The combination often works best.

Who Gets RLS

- Women with heavy periods (losing blood monthly)
- Pregnant women (increased iron needs)
- Vegetarians and vegans (plant iron absorbs poorly)
- Anyone with digestive problems affecting absorption
- People on PPIs or H2 blockers long-term (block iron absorption)
- Older adults (decreased absorption with age)

Chronic Muscle Tension: The Switch That Won't Turn Off

Maybe your problem isn't cramps or restless legs. Maybe it's that your neck and shoulders are always tight. Your jaw clenches. Your back aches constantly. You've tried stretching, massage, physical therapy. Nothing provides lasting relief.

This is The Muscle Switch stuck in the ON position—not dramatically enough to cramp, but enough that your muscles never fully release.

The culprit is usually the calcium-magnesium balance. You might be getting plenty of calcium (dairy, supplements) but not enough magnesium to balance it. Your muscles receive the "contract" signal but can't hear the "relax" signal clearly.

The Nervous System Connection

Chronic tension also connects to Chapter 5. When your nervous system is stuck in fight-or-flight, your muscles stay tense as part of the stress response. Addressing minerals helps, but if trauma or chronic stress is driving your nervous system dysregulation, you'll need both approaches.

Safety Check: When to See a Doctor

Stop reading and see a doctor TODAY if you have:

- Sudden severe pain that doesn't resolve
- Muscle weakness that's getting progressively worse
- Chest pain or difficulty breathing
- Numbness or tingling spreading from one area to others
- Loss of bowel or bladder control
- Severe pain with fever

See a doctor this week if:

- Pain is severe, persistent, or worsening despite rest
- Cramps happen during the day with activity (not just at night)
- Muscle weakness interferes with daily activities
- Restless legs don't improve after several months of addressing iron and magnesium

Conditions minerals won't fix:

- Pinched nerves, herniated discs, spinal stenosis
- Peripheral artery disease, blood clots
- Neuropathy from diabetes or other causes
- Medication side effects (especially statins)
- Fibromyalgia, chronic fatigue syndrome

If you're not sure: Does rest make it better? (Good sign—probably not serious.) Is it getting worse over time? (Red flag—get evaluated.)

Feel—Pause—Act: Before You Do Anything

You just read a lot of information. If you're in chronic pain or haven't slept well in months, your brain is probably racing right now.

Before you act, check in with yourself.

FEEL: Notice what's happening

Is your heart racing? Are you making a mental shopping list of supplements? If yes, you're activated. Decisions made while activated usually backfire.

PAUSE: Don't act yet

Close this book. Take three slow breaths. Step away for ten minutes. The information will still be here. Your muscle problems took months or years to develop. They'll take time to address properly. There's no deadline.

ACT: Once you're calmer

Come back when you can think clearly. Then take ONE step: make a doctor's appointment, or start tracking your symptoms, or add magnesium-rich foods to your diet. One step. One change. One conversation at a time.

Working with Your Doctor

This section gives you what you need for an informed conversation with your healthcare provider. The specific plan for YOUR body needs to come from someone who knows your full health picture.

Where to start: Your primary care doctor can order testing and provide initial treatment. If problems don't respond, consider a sports medicine doctor (if you're athletic), a functional medicine doctor (for comprehensive mineral assessment), or a neurologist (for severe RLS).

Tier 1: Start Here

For cramps and muscle tension—discuss magnesium

What to say:

"I'm having frequent muscle cramps [or chronic tension]. Research shows magnesium is required for muscle relaxation—it's literally the 'off switch' for muscle contraction. What do you think about trying supplementation?"

Questions to ask:

- Which form do you recommend? I've read that glycinate and malate absorb better than oxide.
- What dose should I start with?
- Are there any interactions with my current medications?
- How long should I try this before we reassess?

What to track:

Frequency and severity of cramps (rate 1–10), time of day they occur, sleep quality, any digestive side effects, how consistently you're taking it.

Timeline: Many people notice improvement within 1–2 weeks. Give it 6–8 weeks for full assessment.

For restless legs—get ferritin tested

What to say:

"I have restless legs that are affecting my sleep. Research shows RLS symptoms often improve significantly when ferritin is above 75 ng/mL, not just above the lab minimum of 15. Can we check my ferritin specifically?"

Questions to ask:

- What's my actual ferritin number? (Not just "normal" or "fine")
- If I supplement, when should we retest?
- Should I take it with vitamin C? What should I avoid taking it with?
- Could any of my current medications be affecting iron absorption?

What to track:

RLS symptom frequency (nights per week), severity (1–10), how long symptoms last, sleep quality, any side effects from iron (constipation is common).

Timeline: Iron repletion is slow. Expect 8–12 weeks minimum before significant improvement. Some people feel somewhat better before ferritin fully normalizes; others need to reach 75+ before symptoms resolve.

Tier 2: If Tier 1 Doesn't Work

If you've tried magnesium for cramps and it hasn't helped after 6–8 weeks: Is absorption an issue? (Chapter 7—gut health affects mineral absorption) Is your nervous system driving the tension? (Chapter 5—chronic stress keeps muscles contracted) Are there structural issues that need physical therapy? Would a different form of magnesium work better?

If you've tried iron for RLS and it hasn't helped: Is ferritin actually rising on retesting? (If not, you have an absorption issue) Have you given it enough time? (Iron repletion takes months, not weeks) Do you need magnesium as well? (Many people need both) Is there ongoing blood loss keeping ferritin low? (Heavy periods, GI issues)

When to Push Back or Get a Second Opinion

Your doctor should take you seriously if: symptoms significantly affect your sleep or daily life, you have risk factors (heavy periods, vegetarian diet, digestive disorders, medications that deplete minerals), you've tried their initial recommendations without improvement.

Red flags in doctor responses: "It's just aging" (without any investigation). "Your tests are normal" (without telling you the actual numbers). Prescribing medication for symptoms without investigating cause.

You deserve clear explanations and partnership in your care.

Special Situations

Pregnancy
Leg cramps are extremely common. Magnesium supplementation often helps and is safe at appropriate doses. Work with your OB.

Over 65
Absorption decreases with age. You may need higher doses or different forms. More frequent monitoring is appropriate.

Kidney Disease
Your kidneys regulate mineral balance. Do NOT supplement potassium without medical supervision. Magnesium also needs closer monitoring. Work with your nephrologist.

Multiple Medications

Many deplete minerals. Bring your complete medication list to appointments. Ask specifically: "Could any of these be causing or worsening my symptoms?"

What Success Looks Like

Magnesium for cramps: Many people notice improvement within 1–2 weeks. Full effect may take 4–6 weeks.

Iron for RLS: This takes longer. Ferritin rises slowly—expect 8–12 weeks minimum before significant improvement. Some people notice changes before ferritin fully normalizes; others need to reach 75+ before symptoms resolve.

What improvement looks like: Cramps less frequent (from every night to once a week). Cramps less severe (wake you briefly instead of leaving you hobbling). Restless legs symptoms reduced (can fall asleep, stay asleep longer). Chronic tension releasing (shoulders not at your ears all day).

You're looking for progress, not perfection. Most people won't have complete elimination of all symptoms, but significant improvement in quality of life.

Protection—Safety—Healing Check-in

You just learned about muscle function and minerals. Before you move on, notice where you are.

Feeling overwhelmed? This was a lot?

That's okay. Here's the simple version: Magnesium for cramps. Ferritin above 75 for restless legs. That's it for now. Pick one thing. Make one appointment. Don't try to fix everything at once.

Feeling stable? Ready to take action?

Good. You understand The Muscle Switch. Start tracking your symptoms this week. Make an appointment to discuss magnesium or get ferritin tested. Bring the specific questions from this chapter.

Feeling engaged? Want the full picture?

Excellent. Request comprehensive testing (RBC magnesium, ferritin, potassium). Consider whether nervous system work (Chapter 5) or gut healing (Chapter 7) might be affecting your muscles too. Build the whole system.

The Bottom Line

Your muscles speak through cramps, restless legs, and chronic tension.

They're telling you The Muscle Switch isn't working properly.

CALCIUM turns muscles ON

MAGNESIUM turns them OFF

POTASSIUM keeps the switch working

IRON wires the whole system

You now know what to ask for. Make the appointment. Request the tests. Have the conversation.

Your muscles have been trying to tell you something. Now you know how to listen.

→ *Coming up in Chapter 9: If muscle cramps wake you at night, you already know sleep is suffering. But what if your problem isn't cramps—what if you just can't fall asleep, or you wake at 3 AM and can't get back to sleep, or you sleep 8 hours and wake up exhausted? The next chapter tackles sleep directly, and you'll see The Muscle Switch show up again—because magnesium's role in helping you relax doesn't stop at your muscles.*

CHAPTER 9

Sleep: When Your Body Won't Rest

You're so tired, but sleep won't come

Eleven at night. You're exhausted. You've been tired all day. You finally get into bed, close your eyes, and... nothing.

Your body is tired, but your brain won't shut off. Your mind races. You're thinking about work, replaying conversations, making lists. An hour passes. Then two. You're still awake, getting more frustrated by the minute.

Or maybe you fall asleep fine, but you wake at 3 AM. Your eyes snap open. You're fully awake. Your mind starts spinning. You try to go back to sleep. You can't.

Or maybe you sleep eight hours. Your tracker says you slept great. But you wake up feeling like you were hit by a truck. You're not refreshed. Nobody believes you because "you got plenty of sleep."

So you talked to your doctor. They told you: "Try melatonin." "Reduce screen time." "Practice good sleep hygiene." "Everyone has trouble sleeping sometimes." Maybe they prescribed sleeping pills that made you groggy or stopped working. Maybe they said waking at 3 AM is just what happens as you age.

You left feeling dismissed.

Here's what nobody told you: Your body needs specific minerals to sleep. Your brain needs magnesium to produce calming neurotransmitters. You need iron for oxygen delivery and deep sleep. When these minerals run low, your body literally cannot sleep properly—no matter how tired you are, no matter how good your sleep hygiene is.

Standard blood work doesn't check for this. Doctors aren't trained to connect sleep problems with mineral deficiency. So you suffer while the real problem goes untreated.

They Said It Was Just Stress—They Were Wrong

"Just stress." "Just anxiety." "Just aging." "You need to relax more."

TRUTH: Magnesium deficiency causes insomnia. Research shows magnesium activates your parasympathetic nervous system—your "rest and digest" mode. It increases GABA, the neurotransmitter that calms your brain. It regulates melatonin production. Studies show magnesium supplementation improves both sleep quality and sleep duration. But doctors rarely check magnesium for sleep problems. They prescribe sleeping pills instead.

TRUTH: Low iron disrupts sleep quality. Your brain needs iron for proper oxygen delivery during sleep. People with low ferritin—even in the "normal" range—report poor sleep quality, frequent waking, and non-restorative sleep. The same iron deficiency that causes restless legs (Chapter 8) also prevents deep, restorative sleep.

TRUTH: Sleep problems aren't just "bad sleep hygiene." You can have perfect sleep hygiene—dark room, cool temperature, no screens—and still not sleep if your body doesn't have the minerals it needs.

This isn't your fault. It's biochemistry.

Your Brain Has an OFF Switch Too

Remember The Muscle Switch from Chapter 8? Calcium turns muscles ON, magnesium turns them OFF. When magnesium is low, your muscles cramp because they're stuck in the ON position.

Your brain works the same way.

When Magnesium Is Adequate

Your brain can shift from "active and alert" to "calm and ready for sleep."

GABA—your brain's calming neurotransmitter—increases.

Your parasympathetic nervous system engages.

Your thoughts slow down.

Sleep comes.

When Magnesium Is Low

Your brain's OFF switch is broken.

Your nervous system stays in GO mode.

Your thoughts keep firing.

You're exhausted but your mind won't stop.

Sleep becomes impossible.

This is why lying there trying harder to sleep doesn't work. You can't willpower your way past a broken switch.

The Sleep Cascade

Magnesium → increases GABA (calms brain) → activates parasympathetic nervous system (rest mode) → enables melatonin production → allows sleep

Break any link in that chain, and sleep suffers.

Iron's Role

Iron carries oxygen to your brain during sleep. When iron is low, oxygen delivery is compromised. Your sleep becomes fragmented. You don't reach deep stages. You wake frequently. You don't feel restored even after eight hours.

The Vicious Cycle

Poor sleep depletes minerals. Mineral deficiency causes poor sleep.

When you don't sleep well:

- Stress hormones stay elevated (burning through magnesium)
- Your body can't restore depleted minerals (restoration happens during deep sleep)
- Inflammation increases (depleting zinc and other minerals)

Breaking it requires addressing both sleep and minerals simultaneously.

The Four Types of Sleep Problems

Not all sleep problems are the same. Your pattern gives clues about what's wrong—and what to discuss with your doctor.

1. Can't Fall Asleep

You're exhausted. You get into bed. You lie there for an hour, two hours. Your mind won't shut off. Your body feels tired but wired.

What's Happening

Your brain's OFF switch isn't working. Your nervous system is stuck in fight-or-flight mode (Chapter 5). Magnesium is too low to produce adequate GABA or shift you into rest mode.

Research shows: Magnesium supplementation consistently improves sleep onset time—people fall asleep faster when magnesium levels are adequate.

What to discuss with your doctor:

"I can't fall asleep for 1–2 hours most nights even when exhausted. Research shows magnesium helps with sleep onset. Can we try this?"

- Which form would you recommend—glycinate or threonate?
- Should we also evaluate for anxiety? (Anxiety commonly causes sleep onset problems and may need additional treatment)

What to track: How long it takes to fall asleep, what your mind does (racing thoughts? worry?), whether you feel physically tense or relaxed.

Timeline: Many people notice improvement within 1–2 weeks. Give it 6–8 weeks for full assessment.

2. Wake in the Middle of the Night

You fall asleep fine. Then you wake up—often around the same time every night, frequently 2–4 AM. You're fully awake. You lie there for hours.

What's Happening

This pattern usually involves cortisol dysregulation or blood sugar crashes—both connected to magnesium. Cortisol should be at its lowest point around midnight to 1 AM. But when your system is dysregulated—

often from chronic stress burning through magnesium—cortisol spikes when it should be silent. Your body thinks there's danger. You wake up. Low magnesium also affects blood sugar. When blood sugar drops too low overnight, your body releases cortisol and adrenaline to raise it—which wakes you up.

What to discuss with your doctor:

"I wake at [specific time] almost every night and can't get back to sleep. Could this be cortisol or blood sugar related?"

- Would magnesium help regulate this?
- Should we test cortisol rhythm?
- Could this be hormonal? (For women in perimenopause—night sweats commonly cause this pattern)

What to track: Exact time you wake, what you notice when you wake (anxious? hot? heart racing?), whether the pattern is consistent.

Timeline: Sleep maintenance often takes longer to improve—potentially several weeks to months.

3. Restless Sleep / Tossing and Turning

You're asleep, but not really. You toss and turn all night. You never feel like you've slept deeply. Your tracker shows lots of light sleep, minimal deep sleep.

What's Happening

Your muscles aren't relaxing properly (The Muscle Switch from Chapter 8—magnesium deficiency). Or your oxygen delivery is impaired (iron deficiency), keeping you in lighter sleep stages.

Research shows: Magnesium improves sleep quality and increases time in deep sleep. Iron repletion improves subjective sleep quality even without diagnosed restless legs.

What to discuss with your doctor:

"I toss and turn all night and never reach deep sleep. Could magnesium or iron be contributing?"

- Can we check ferritin? Research shows low-normal ferritin affects sleep quality.
- Do I need a sleep study to rule out apnea? (Apnea also causes fragmented sleep)

What to track: Whether you're aware of restlessness or partner reports it, any leg discomfort, what your sleep tracker shows.

Timeline: Magnesium may help within 1–2 weeks. Iron takes much longer (8–12 weeks for significant improvement).

4. Sleep but Don't Feel Rested

You sleep eight or nine hours. But you wake up exhausted. Nobody believes you because "you got plenty of sleep."

What's Happening

You're not reaching deep, restorative sleep stages. This can be minerals (magnesium, iron), but it can also be sleep apnea, depression, chronic pain, or medications.

What to discuss with your doctor:

"I sleep 8–9 hours but wake exhausted. What could cause this?"

- Do I need a sleep study? (Describe any snoring, gasping, witnessed breathing pauses)
- Should we screen for depression? (Common cause of non-restorative sleep)
- Could my medications be affecting sleep quality?

What to track: Hours slept, snoring (ask partner), morning headaches, falling asleep during the day, mood.

Timeline: This is complex. May require sleep study, mental health evaluation, AND mineral assessment. Work with your doctor systematically.

Critical: If you snore loudly, gasp during sleep, or your partner notices you stop breathing—you need a sleep study before assuming it's minerals. Sleep apnea causes non-restorative sleep and is dangerous if untreated. No amount of magnesium will fix it.

Safety Check: When Sleep Problems Need Medical Evaluation

See a doctor THIS WEEK if:

- Loud snoring with gasping or pauses in breathing (sleep apnea can be life-threatening)
- Thoughts of harming yourself (sleep deprivation can trigger suicidal thoughts—this is an emergency)
- Severe insomnia affecting your ability to function safely
- Hallucinations or severe confusion from sleep deprivation

See a doctor soon if:

- Chronic insomnia (most nights for 3+ months) affecting quality of life
- You fall asleep unintentionally during the day
- You've tried addressing minerals and sleep hygiene for 2–3 months with no improvement

Conditions minerals won't fix:

- Sleep apnea (needs CPAP or other treatment)
- Narcolepsy (needs medical treatment)
- Circadian rhythm disorders (may need light therapy)
- Depression or anxiety disorders (need mental health treatment—minerals are supportive, not primary)
- Medication-induced sleep problems (discuss with prescribing doctor)

When in doubt, get evaluated. Sleep apnea especially is dangerous if missed.

What Your Doctor Probably Doesn't Know

About magnesium:

"Normal" serum magnesium doesn't predict sleep quality—most magnesium is inside cells. RBC magnesium is more accurate but rarely ordered. Magnesium glycinate works best for sleep (oxide absorbs poorly, citrate causes diarrhea). Timing matters—take at bedtime.

About iron:

Low ferritin affects sleep even without restless legs. Lab "normal" starts at 15, but many people need ferritin above 50–75 for optimal sleep. People suffer with ferritin of 25 while doctors say "fine."

About melatonin supplements:

They don't work well if mineral balance is off. Fix the underlying deficiency first.

About sleep hygiene:

It helps, but perfect sleep hygiene won't override mineral deficiency. Doctors often stop at sleep hygiene education without investigating biochemical causes.

Feel—Pause—Act: Before You Do Anything

Remember Feel-Pause-Act from Chapter 8? It applies here too—especially because sleep deprivation impairs judgment.

If you're exhausted and desperate, if you're planning to buy five supplements tonight, if you're thinking "I need to fix this RIGHT NOW"—

PAUSE

Sleep problems took time to develop. They'll take time to address properly. Decisions made while sleep-deprived usually backfire.

Come back to this chapter tomorrow, after you've rested. Take ONE step: make a doctor's appointment, or start tracking your sleep. One step at a time.

If you're in crisis:

If you haven't slept more than 2–3 hours per night for over a week, if you're having thoughts of self-harm, if you can't function safely—call your doctor today. You might need short-term medication to break the cycle while you investigate root causes.

Working with Your Doctor

Your primary care doctor can order testing and provide initial treatment. Here's what to discuss:

For any sleep problem:

- Request magnesium trial (glycinate form, taken at bedtime)
- Request ferritin testing if sleep is non-restorative or restless
- Discuss whether sleep study is warranted
- Review all medications for sleep effects

Testing to consider:

- Ferritin (goal: above 50–75, not just "above 15")
- RBC magnesium if available (more accurate than serum)
- Thyroid function (both hypo and hyper affect sleep)
- Sleep study if any apnea risk factors

When Tier 1 Doesn't Work

If you've tried magnesium, addressed iron if low, ruled out apnea, and still aren't sleeping:

Check absorption (Chapter 7)

If your gut can't absorb minerals, supplements won't help. Signs: digestive issues, long-term PPI use, levels not rising despite supplementation.

Check nervous system (Chapter 5)

If your nervous system is stuck in survival mode from trauma or chronic stress, minerals alone won't override it. You need both.

Consider CBT-I

Cognitive Behavioral Therapy for Insomnia is highly effective for chronic insomnia—often more effective than medication. Ask your doctor for a referral.

What to Track

Keep it simple. Two weeks before your appointment:

Daily

- Bedtime and approximate time you fell asleep
- Number of awakenings
- Total sleep time
- How rested you feel (1–10)
- Caffeine and alcohol

If Supplementing

- What you're taking (specific form)
- Dose and timing
- Any changes in sleep

Bring this to your appointment. It helps your doctor see patterns.

What Success Looks Like

Realistic targets:

- Falling asleep within 20–30 minutes
- Waking 0–1 times briefly
- 7–9 hours total
- Waking reasonably refreshed
- Functioning well during the day

You're looking for significant improvement, not perfection. Most people won't have perfect sleep every night.

Timelines:

- Magnesium: some notice improvement within days; most within 1–2 weeks; full benefits 4–6 weeks
- Iron: 8–12 weeks for significant improvement (ferritin rises slowly)
- CBT-I: typically 4–8 weeks

Protection—Safety—Healing Check-in

You just learned about sleep and minerals. Before you move on, notice where you are.

Exhausted right now? Can barely focus?

That's okay. You don't need to do anything tonight. Here's the simple version: Magnesium glycinate at bedtime. That's it for now. Make one appointment. Rest first, then come back to this chapter.

Functioning but struggling? Ready to take action?

Good. You understand the Sleep Cascade. Identify your type (1–4). Start tracking your sleep this week. Make an appointment to discuss magnesium or get ferritin tested. Bring the specific questions from this chapter.

Stable enough to optimize?

Excellent. Request comprehensive testing (ferritin, RBC magnesium, thyroid). Rule out sleep apnea if any risk factors. Consider whether nervous system work (Chapter 5) or gut healing (Chapter 7) might be affecting your sleep too. Build the whole system.

The Bottom Line

Your brain has an OFF switch, just like your muscles. When magnesium is low, that switch is broken. Your brain can't shift from GO mode to REST mode. Sleep becomes impossible no matter how tired you are.

The Sleep Cascade:

Magnesium → GABA → parasympathetic activation → melatonin → sleep. Break any link, and you lie awake at 2 AM wondering why you can't sleep.

The 3 AM wake-up? Usually cortisol spiking when it should be silent. Magnesium helps regulate that rhythm.

The non-restorative sleep? Rule out apnea first. Then investigate iron, magnesium, depression.

You now know what to ask for. Magnesium glycinate at bedtime. Ferritin above 50–75. The right tests, the right targets, the right conversations.

Your body has been trying to tell you why it can't rest. Now you know how to listen.

→ *Coming up in Chapter 10: If poor sleep is leaving you exhausted, you already know what energy depletion feels like. But what if you're sleeping adequately and still can barely function? What if you need three cups of coffee just to make it through? The next chapter tackles energy and fatigue directly—why iron deficiency causes exhaustion that sleep can't fix.*

CHAPTER 10

Energy and Fatigue

When you can't keep going

It's 2 PM. You slept seven hours last night. You've had coffee. You've eaten lunch. And you're so tired you can barely keep your eyes open.

Not sleepy-tired. Bone-deep, crushing exhaustion. Like your body weighs a thousand pounds. Like every movement requires enormous effort.

You have five more hours of work. Kids to pick up. Dinner to make. But you don't know how you're going to make it.

So you have more coffee. You push through. Tomorrow will be better. But tomorrow isn't better. And the day after that. And the day after that.

You're tired all the time. You wake up tired. You're too tired to exercise, too tired to see friends, too tired to do anything except survive. Your life has shrunk to: work, basic necessities, collapse.

You went to your doctor. They ran blood work. Everything looks "normal." They suggested: "Try exercising more." "Reduce stress." "Maybe you're depressed." "Everyone's tired these days."

You left feeling dismissed. Like you're supposed to just accept that this is your life now.

Here's what nobody told you: Your body needs specific minerals to make energy. At a cellular level, your mitochondria—the power plants in every cell—need iron, magnesium, and other minerals to produce ATP (the energy molecule your body runs on). When these minerals run low, your cells literally cannot make adequate energy. No matter how much you sleep. No matter how hard you try.

They Said It Was Just Being Tired—They Were Wrong

Iron deficiency causes fatigue even when you're not anemic.

You can have "normal" hemoglobin but low ferritin (iron stores), and this causes profound exhaustion. Your cells need iron to use oxygen for energy production. When iron stores are low, oxygen delivery is impaired. You're breathing fine, but your cells are starving.

Magnesium deficiency causes fatigue at the cellular level.

Every cell needs magnesium to make ATP—the energy molecule that powers everything. When magnesium is low, your mitochondria can't efficiently convert food into energy. You're exhausted no matter how much you rest.

Your thyroid might be "normal" but not optimal.

Doctors check TSH. If it's in range, they say your thyroid is fine. But zinc and selenium are required to convert T4 to T3 (the active form). You can have "normal" TSH but impaired conversion—and crushing fatigue.

About thyroid minerals:

Throughout this book, when we discuss thyroid testing and support, we mention selenium and zinc — the two minerals most often discussed in functional thyroid care. But thyroid function actually depends on four minerals working together:

- **Iodine** — the substrate your thyroid uses to make hormones (T4 contains four iodine atoms; T3 contains three)
- **Selenium** — required for the deiodinase enzymes that convert T4 to active T3, and for protecting the thyroid from oxidative damage
- **Zinc** — required for T4-to-T3 conversion and for thyroid hormone receptor function
- **Iron** — required by thyroid peroxidase (TPO), the enzyme that builds thyroid hormones in the first place

The US population overall is considered iodine-sufficient by median intake. But that median masks a real problem in women specifically. Recent NHANES data (2017–2018) show 24% of US females aged 14 and older have inadequate iodine intake — double the rate from 2001–2002. Among women of reproductive age, 35% are below the estimated average requirement. Among pregnant women, 46% are. The trend has been worsening for two decades.

Why? Reduced iodine content in dairy (industry changes), increased use of non-iodized salt in processed foods, and public health recommendations to lower sodium intake. Sea salt, kosher salt, and Himalayan pink salt are not iodized.

If you have thyroid symptoms with "normal" labs, ask about iodine status — not just selenium and zinc.

Chronic fatigue isn't laziness. Your body is trying to conserve energy because it doesn't have the biochemical resources to make more. This is physiology, not character.

Your Cells Are Power Plants

Remember The Muscle Switch from Chapters 8 and 9? Now extend that concept to every cell in your body.

Each cell contains mitochondria—tiny power plants that convert food and oxygen into ATP, the energy currency that powers everything you do. Thinking. Moving. Digesting. Healing. Every single function requires ATP.

The Energy Equation

IRON = FUEL DELIVERY

Carries oxygen in blood. Oxygen is what mitochondria burn to make ATP. **Low iron = cells starving for oxygen.**

MAGNESIUM = THE GENERATOR

Required to actually make ATP. The molecule is Mg-ATP (magnesium bound to ATP). **No magnesium = generator can't run.**

ZINC + SELENIUM = THE THERMOSTAT

Convert thyroid hormone to active form, setting metabolic rate. **Low = metabolism sluggish.**

When any of these run low, your power plants can't produce adequate energy. You're exhausted not because you need more willpower—but because your cells literally can't make the ATP you need to function.

The Vicious Cycle

When you're exhausted, you move less, eat worse, sleep poorly, feel more stressed. Each of these depletes more minerals, which worsens fatigue, which perpetuates the cycle.

Breaking it requires addressing minerals alongside sleep (Chapter 9), nervous system regulation (Chapter 5), and gut health (Chapter 7). But minerals are often the missing piece that makes everything else work.

THE FATIGUE YOUR DOCTOR MISSED

If you're exhausted and your doctor said "your iron is fine," ask one question:

"What was my ferritin?"

Doctors check hemoglobin. If it's normal, they say you're not anemic. Case closed. But ferritin—your iron stores—can be 20, 25, 30. Technically "normal" (lab ranges start at 15). And you're crushed with fatigue because your cells are starving for iron even though you're not anemic.

Research shows people with ferritin below 50 report severe fatigue, reduced exercise capacity, and difficulty concentrating—even with normal hemoglobin.

The Number

Ferritin above 50

Many people need 75–100 to feel normal

If your ferritin is below 50 and you're exhausted, you likely have your answer. Ask your doctor about iron supplementation.

This single test has explained years of unexplained fatigue for people whose doctors never thought to check it.

The Three Types of Fatigue

Your pattern gives clues about what's wrong.

1. Can't Get Started (Morning Fatigue)

You wake exhausted after 7–8 hours of sleep. It takes hours to feel functional. You need multiple cups of coffee to get moving. Mornings are torture.

What's Probably Happening

Cortisol should be highest in the morning—that's what gives you energy to start the day. When cortisol rhythm is disrupted (often from chronic stress depleting magnesium), you wake with low cortisol and feel terrible. This can also indicate suboptimal thyroid function—even "normal" TSH with low Free T3 causes morning fatigue.

What to discuss with your doctor:

"I wake exhausted no matter how much I sleep. Could this be cortisol dysregulation or thyroid-related?"

"Can we check Free T3 and Free T4, not just TSH?"

"Would cortisol testing be useful?"

For a more complete picture, ask about a four-point salivary cortisol test (waking, around 11 AM, around 4 PM, and bedtime). This shows your daily cortisol rhythm rather than a single snapshot. The salivary cortisol test itself is a standard tool in endocrinology — late-night salivary cortisol is a validated screening test for Cushing's syndrome. What's not validated is the "adrenal fatigue" diagnosis that some practitioners build on cortisol-rhythm patterns; mainstream endocrinology doesn't recognize adrenal fatigue as a discrete condition. Even so, the rhythm itself is real biology, and seeing it can be useful information. If your conventional doctor declines and the symptoms warrant it, integrative medicine practitioners and direct-to-consumer functional labs offer the four-point test.

"Could magnesium help regulate cortisol rhythm?"

2. Afternoon Crash

Mornings are okay. Then around 1–3 PM, you crash hard. Overwhelming exhaustion. Can barely function. By evening you might get a second wind, or just stay exhausted.

What's Probably Happening

After eating, blood sugar rises then drops. If magnesium is low (required for proper insulin function), this drop is more dramatic—causing the classic post-lunch crash. Or your mitochondria are struggling: you start the day with whatever energy reserves you have, but by afternoon they're depleted.

What to discuss with your doctor:

"I crash hard every afternoon. Could this be blood sugar or mitochondrial function?"

"Should we check magnesium and fasting glucose/HbA1c?"

"Would magnesium supplementation help stabilize energy?"

3. Constant Exhaustion

Tired when you wake. Tired all day. No good time. Everything feels like pushing through mud. Even 8–10 hours of sleep doesn't help.

What's Probably Happening

This is the most severe pattern. Often indicates multiple mineral deficiencies (iron, magnesium, zinc, B vitamins all low), significant sleep disorders, or serious medical conditions. This pattern requires thorough medical investigation. Don't assume it's just minerals.

What to discuss with your doctor:

"I'm exhausted constantly—no relief from sleep. I need comprehensive investigation."

"Can we check ferritin, magnesium, B12, vitamin D, and full thyroid panel?"

"Do I need a sleep study to rule out apnea?"

"Should we screen for autoimmune conditions or other serious causes?"

Safety Check: When Fatigue Needs Urgent Evaluation

Emergency—go now if:

- Sudden severe fatigue with chest pain, shortness of breath, or irregular heartbeat
- Sudden fatigue with severe headache, confusion, or one-sided weakness
- Thoughts of harming yourself

See a doctor THIS WEEK if:

- New severe fatigue that's rapidly worsening
- Fatigue with unexplained weight loss (10+ pounds)
- Fatigue with fever or night sweats
- Fatigue preventing you from working or caring for yourself

Conditions minerals won't fix:

- Severe anemia (needs diagnosis and treatment)
- Sleep apnea (needs CPAP—if you snore/gasp, get a sleep study first)
- Diabetes (needs blood sugar management)
- Autoimmune diseases (lupus, rheumatoid arthritis, Hashimoto's)
- Depression (real medical condition needing treatment—though minerals may help alongside)
- Chronic Fatigue Syndrome/ME (needs specialized management)
- Cancer or chronic infections

When in doubt, get evaluated. Fatigue can signal serious illness.

What Your Doctor Probably Doesn't Know

About iron:

Research shows iron deficiency without anemia causes significant fatigue. Iron supplementation improves fatigue when ferritin is below 50—even with normal hemoglobin. Yet doctors routinely check only hemoglobin, miss low ferritin, and say "iron is fine."

About magnesium:

Magnesium is required for ATP synthesis. Deficiency impairs mitochondrial function. But serum testing is unreliable (most magnesium is inside cells), so doctors rarely investigate it for fatigue.

About thyroid:

Selenium and zinc convert T4 to T3 (active form). You can have "normal" TSH but impaired conversion. Doctors rarely check Free T3 or mineral status affecting thyroid function.

About "normal" ranges:

Lab ranges show what 95% of people have, not what's optimal. Many people feel terrible at the low end of "normal." Ferritin of 20 is "normal" but often causes significant fatigue.

Feel—Pause—Act: Before You Do Anything

Remember Feel-Pause-Act from Chapters 8 and 9? It applies here too.

If you've been exhausted for months and finally see a possible answer, your brain wants to FIX IT NOW. You're planning to buy iron and magnesium tonight, start everything tomorrow, feel better by next week.

PAUSE

Fatigue that developed over months won't resolve overnight. Iron repletion takes 3–6 months. Decisions made while exhausted usually backfire—you try everything at once, can't tell what's working, quit when results aren't immediate.

Take ONE step: make a doctor's appointment and request ferritin testing. One step at a time.

If you're in crisis:

If you literally cannot work or care for yourself, call your doctor today. You may need urgent evaluation and short-term support while investigating causes.

Working with Your Doctor

Your primary care doctor can order testing and provide initial treatment.

Essential Tests to Request

Ferritin (not just hemoglobin)

"Research shows ferritin below 50 causes fatigue even without anemia. Can we check this specifically?"

Full thyroid panel (TSH, Free T3, Free T4)

"Can we check Free T3, not just TSH? Conversion problems cause fatigue even with normal TSH."

Magnesium (RBC if available)

"Can we check magnesium? I know serum isn't perfect, but if it's low, that's useful."

Vitamin D and B12

Both deficiencies cause fatigue and are common.

When Results Come Back

Don't accept "everything's normal." Get actual numbers.

"What's my ferritin level?" (Goal: above 50, ideally 75–100)

"What's my Free T3?" (Not just "thyroid is fine")

"Where do I fall in each range—low end, middle, or high?"

If you're at the low end of "normal": "Research shows many people feel better with levels in the mid-to-upper range. Can we try supplementation?"

If Ferritin Is Low

Iron supplementation typically 65–200 mg elemental iron daily—ask your doctor about the right dose and form for you. Forms matter:

Ferrous bisglycinate / iron glycinate

Better absorbed, fewer GI side effects

Ferrous sulfate

Cheapest but often causes constipation

- Take with vitamin C (enhances absorption)
- Avoid taking with calcium, coffee, tea (block absorption)
- Expect dark stools (normal)
- Retest in 8–12 weeks

Timeline: Iron repletion takes 3–6 months. You may feel somewhat better before ferritin fully normalizes, but patience is required.

If Magnesium Is Low or Symptoms Suggest Deficiency

Magnesium supplementation typically 200–400 mg daily.

- Magnesium glycinate: well absorbed, good for energy
- Magnesium malate: may be particularly good for fatigue
- Avoid magnesium oxide: poorly absorbed

Some people notice improvement within days to weeks.

When First-Line Approaches Don't Work

You've tested, supplemented appropriately, given it adequate time. Still exhausted.

Check absorption (Chapter 7)

If your gut can't absorb nutrients, supplements won't help. Signs: digestive issues, PPI use, levels not rising on retest despite supplementing.

Check nervous system (Chapter 5)

Chronic fight-or-flight burns through minerals and prioritizes survival over energy production. If trauma or chronic stress is driving your system, minerals alone won't override it.

Check sleep (Chapter 9)

Sleep apnea causes crushing fatigue that minerals won't fix. If you snore or gasp, get a sleep study.

Consider conditions minerals won't fix

ME/CFS, fibromyalgia, autoimmune diseases, chronic infections. These need specialized diagnosis and treatment. It's okay to accept that minerals aren't your answer and pursue proper diagnosis for your actual condition.

What to Track

Two weeks before your appointment:

Daily

- Energy level: morning, afternoon, evening (1–10 scale)
- Sleep hours and quality
- Caffeine intake
- Any patterns (worse certain days? after certain activities?)

If Supplementing

- What you're taking, dose, consistency
- Any changes in energy
- Any side effects

Bring this data to your appointment.

What Success Looks Like

Realistic Timelines

- Magnesium: days to weeks for some people
- Iron: 3–6 months (may feel somewhat better before ferritin normalizes)
- Vitamin D: 6–8 weeks
- B12: days to weeks with injections, longer oral

What Improvement Looks Like

- Waking with energy more often
- Getting through the day without crashing
- Able to exercise or be more active
- Improved concentration
- Able to engage in life again

You're aiming for functional energy—not perfection. Everyone has tired days. The goal is consistent, adequate energy to live your life.

Protection—Safety—Healing Check-in

You just learned about energy and minerals. Before you move on, notice where you are.

So exhausted you can barely process this?

That's okay. Here's the simple version: Get ferritin tested. That's it for now. Make one appointment. Ask for one test. Rest first, then come back to this chapter.

Tired but functional? Ready to investigate?

Good. You understand your cells are power plants. Identify your fatigue type (1–3). Start tracking your energy this week. Make an appointment for comprehensive testing—ferritin, thyroid panel, magnesium, B12, vitamin D.

Stable enough to optimize your energy?

Excellent. Request full testing including RBC magnesium and Free T3. Consider whether nervous system work (Chapter 5), gut healing (Chapter 7), or sleep optimization (Chapter 9) might be limiting your energy too. Build the whole system.

The Bottom Line

Your cells are power plants. Iron delivers the oxygen they burn. Magnesium runs the generator that makes ATP. When either runs low, the lights go out.

You're not tired because you're lazy or need more will power. You're tired because your cells can't make energy.

The test your doctor probably skipped: **Ferritin**

The mineral that powers everything: **Magnesium**

You now know what to ask for. Ferritin above 50 (ideally 75–100). Magnesium levels checked. Full thyroid panel including Free T3. The right tests, the right targets, the right conversations.

Your body has been trying to tell you why it can't keep going. Now you know how to listen.

→ *Coming up in Chapter 11: Fatigue affects your body. But what about your brain? What if you can't concentrate, your memory is failing, your mood has crashed? What if anxiety has taken over? The next chapter tackles brain, mood, and mental clarity—why iron affects neurotransmitters, how magnesium regulates your stress response, and how to work with your doctor when your brain isn't working right.*

CHAPTER 11

Brain, Mood, and Mental Clarity

When your mind won't cooperate

You're in a meeting and someone asks you a question. You know the answer. You've known it for years. But the word won't come. It's right there, on the tip of your tongue, and... nothing. You stumble. Everyone stares. The word surfaces ten minutes later when you're alone in the bathroom.

Or maybe it's darker than that. Maybe you wake up and the world feels gray. Not sad, exactly. Just flat. Nothing sounds good. Nothing feels worth doing. You go through the motions but you're not really there.

Or maybe it's the opposite—your mind won't stop. Racing thoughts. Constant worry. Your heart pounds for no reason. You can't relax even when everything is fine.

So you went to your doctor. For the brain fog: "That's normal with stress." "It's just aging." For the mood issues: "Here's an antidepressant." "Try therapy." "Everyone feels anxious sometimes."

Maybe the antidepressant helped. Maybe it didn't. Maybe you've tried multiple medications and nothing works quite right.

Here's what nobody asked you: When's the last time someone checked your iron? Your magnesium? Your zinc?

Probably never.

Your brain is the most metabolically demanding organ in your body—2% of your weight, 20% of your energy. It requires specific minerals to produce neurotransmitters, generate energy, and function properly. When those minerals run low, your brain doesn't work right. No amount of willpower fixes a biochemical problem.

CRITICAL SAFETY INFORMATION—READ THIS FIRST

This chapter requires a different approach than the others.

If you're in crisis right now—stop reading and get help:

988 Suicide and Crisis Lifeline (call or text, 24/7)

911 For immediate danger

Text HOME to 741741 Crisis Text Line

Emergency Room Go immediately if you're in danger

What minerals CANNOT do:

- Cure depression or anxiety
- Replace antidepressants or therapy
- Fix a mental health crisis
- Treat bipolar disorder, schizophrenia, or PTSD

What minerals CAN do:

- Support brain function while you get proper treatment
- Reduce some symptoms if you're deficient
- Potentially help medications work better
- Be one piece of a comprehensive treatment plan

Think of it this way: If your car has a flat tire AND is out of oil, adding oil won't fix the flat tire. But running on no oil will destroy your engine. Minerals are the oil. Therapy and medication (when needed) fix the tire.

Please don't use this chapter to stop taking medication or skip therapy. Use it to ask your doctor about comprehensive evaluation that includes checking mineral status.

They Said It Was Just Depression—They Were Partly Right

"Depression is all in your head—just think positive."

TRUTH: Depression is real. Anxiety is real. These are genuine medical conditions, not character flaws.

"If antidepressants don't work, you're just not trying hard enough."

TRUTH: Sometimes what looks like "treatment-resistant depression" is depression PLUS mineral deficiency—and treating one without the other doesn't work.

"Brain fog is just stress or aging—nothing to do about it."

TRUTH: Sometimes what looks like depression is actually iron deficiency. Sometimes what looks like anxiety is actually magnesium deficiency.

Iron deficiency mimics depression

A woman goes to her doctor—exhausted, unmotivated, can't concentrate, doesn't enjoy anything. She's diagnosed with depression and prescribed an antidepressant. It doesn't really help. Turns out she was severely low in iron.

Iron deficiency and depression look identical: extreme tiredness, trouble thinking, low motivation, feeling emotionally flat, loss of interest. Research shows women with low iron are significantly more likely to experience depression. When iron is corrected, mood often improves.

> This is especially important for women—you lose blood monthly, pregnancy depletes iron dramatically, and you're twice as likely as men to be diagnosed with depression. These facts are connected.

Magnesium deficiency causes anxiety

Magnesium regulates your nervous system's stress response. It increases GABA—the neurotransmitter that calms your brain. When magnesium is low, your nervous system stays activated. You can't calm down even when you're safe.

Remember Chapter 5: When your nervous system is stuck in fight-or-flight, everything feels threatening. Magnesium is one of the key minerals that helps your nervous system regulate.

Zinc deficiency contributes to depression

Zinc is concentrated in brain areas that regulate mood. It's involved in producing serotonin. Research shows people with depression often have lower zinc levels, and zinc supplementation (as an add-on to antidepressants) improves outcomes in some studies.

But—zinc worked as an addition to antidepressants, not a replacement.

Your Brain Runs a Neurotransmitter Factory

Remember the power plants concept from Chapter 10? Your brain is the most demanding power plant in your body. And it runs a neurotransmitter factory that needs specific minerals as raw materials.

IRON → DOPAMINE	MAGNESIUM → GABA	ZINC → SEROTONIN
Motivation and pleasure. The enzyme that makes dopamine requires iron. No iron = no motivation, no pleasure, no focus.	Your brain's calming neurotransmitter. Quiets racing thoughts. No magnesium = anxiety, racing thoughts, can't relax.	The "feel good" neurotransmitter targeted by most antidepressants. No zinc = impaired serotonin = depression.

When raw materials run low, the factory can't produce what you need. You can't think clearly. You can't feel right. And medication alone can't compensate for missing building blocks—it's trying to boost neurotransmitters your brain can't make.

This is why some people try antidepressant after antidepressant without relief. The medication is trying to increase serotonin, but if zinc is low, the brain can't make enough serotonin to increase.

BEFORE THEY CALL IT "TREATMENT-RESISTANT"

If antidepressants aren't working and your doctor is ready to try medication #3 or #4, ask one question:

"Have we checked my ferritin, B12, vitamin D, and zinc?"

A significant percentage of people labeled "treatment-resistant" have undiagnosed nutritional deficiencies. When corrected, treatment response improves.

This testing isn't part of standard psychiatric workups. Psychiatrists aren't trained in nutritional medicine. So people try medication after medication, get labeled "treatment-resistant," and nobody checks if they're missing something basic that their brain needs.

Before trying the next medication, get comprehensive nutritional testing. This single step has helped people who spent years being told nothing would work.

Three Types of Brain Problems

1. Brain Fog and Cognitive Dysfunction

Can't find words. Difficulty concentrating. Reading but not absorbing. Forgetting what you were doing. Mental slowness. Thinking through mud.

What's Probably Happening: Your brain isn't getting what it needs—oxygen (iron), energy (magnesium, B vitamins), or proper signaling (zinc, B12). Thyroid dysfunction also causes brain fog.

> **What to discuss with your doctor:**
>
> **"I have significant brain fog affecting my function. Can we check ferritin, B12, thyroid, and magnesium?"**
>
> ***"Could any of my medications be contributing?"***

Important: Brain fog can also be caused by sleep deprivation (Chapter 9), chronic stress (Chapter 5), gut issues (Chapter 7), medications, autoimmune conditions, hormonal changes, or long COVID. Don't assume it's just minerals.

2. Depression and Low Mood

The world feels gray. Things you used to enjoy don't bring pleasure anymore. You feel empty, hopeless, or numb. Sleep, appetite, or energy have shifted. Getting out of bed feels heavy. Sometimes worse in the morning.

> **Thoughts of death or suicide?**
>
> **This is an emergency—call 988 or go to the ER.**

What's Probably Happening: Depression has multiple causes—genetics, trauma, life circumstances, brain chemistry, and sometimes nutritional deficiency.

Mineral connections: Iron deficiency (low dopamine), zinc deficiency (low serotonin), B12 deficiency (directly causes depression), vitamin D deficiency (strongly associated with depression).

What to discuss with your doctor:

"I've been struggling with depression. Before we adjust medications, can we check ferritin, B12, vitamin D, and zinc to rule out deficiencies?"

"I want comprehensive treatment—therapy, medication if needed, AND addressing any nutritional factors."

Critical: Minerals are ONE factor. Depression typically requires comprehensive treatment—therapy, possibly medication, lifestyle changes, AND addressing deficiencies.

3. Anxiety and Overwhelm

Constant worry. Racing thoughts. Physical symptoms (racing heart, tight chest, trembling). Can't relax even when safe. Panic attacks. Sleep problems.

What's Probably Happening: Your nervous system is stuck in fight-or-flight (Chapter 5). You're perceiving threat even when you're safe.

Mineral connections: Magnesium deficiency (can't produce GABA, can't calm down), zinc-copper imbalance (high copper increases agitation).

What to discuss with your doctor:

"My anxiety isn't responding fully to treatment. Can we check magnesium and look at the zinc-copper ratio?"

"I'm also working on nervous system regulation—would magnesium support that?"

The nervous system connection: If you have significant trauma history, minerals alone won't fix your anxiety. You need nervous system work (Chapter 5) AND addressing deficiencies.

Safety Check: When to Get Help Now

EMERGENCY—call 911 or go to ER:

- Thoughts of hurting yourself or ending your life
- Hearing voices or seeing things that aren't there
- Severe confusion or disorientation
- You've harmed yourself

CALL 988 (Suicide & Crisis Lifeline):

- Thoughts of suicide but not immediate danger
- Need to talk to someone right now
- Emotional crisis

SEE A MENTAL HEALTH PROFESSIONAL THIS WEEK:

- Symptoms affecting ability to work or care for yourself
- Depression or anxiety for more than two weeks
- Current treatment isn't working
- Using alcohol or drugs to cope

What minerals won't fix: Bipolar disorder, schizophrenia, severe PTSD, active addiction, OCD—these need specialized treatment. Minerals support overall brain health but cannot treat these conditions.

What Your Doctor Probably Doesn't Know

About iron: Research shows iron deficiency (low ferritin even without anemia) is associated with depression and cognitive impairment. Yet mental health providers rarely check ferritin.

About magnesium: Studies show magnesium supplementation reduces anxiety in people who are deficient. Yet psychiatrists rarely check magnesium or recommend it for anxiety.

About zinc: Research shows zinc supplementation improves antidepressant response. Yet zinc isn't part of standard depression workups.

About treatment-resistant depression: Before labeling someone treatment-resistant, comprehensive nutritional assessment should be done. It usually isn't.

Feel—Pause—Act: Before You Do Anything

If you've been struggling and this chapter feels like a lifeline, pause.

FEEL:

If you're thinking about stopping your medication to try supplements instead—please don't. Stopping antidepressants suddenly can cause withdrawal and worsening depression.

PAUSE:

If you're thinking about skipping therapy because minerals are the "real" answer—please don't. Minerals are one piece, not the whole picture.

ACT:

The goal is to ADD mineral investigation to your current treatment, not REPLACE your current treatment.

Calm action looks like:

"I'll bring this up with my psychiatrist and ask for comprehensive testing while continuing my current treatment."

Working with Your Doctor

1. Continue your current treatment

Keep taking medication. Keep going to therapy. This chapter is about adding investigation, not abandoning what might be helping.

2. Request comprehensive testing

Say:

"I've been struggling with [depression/anxiety/brain fog] and I'd like to rule out nutritional deficiencies that might be contributing. Can we test ferritin, B12, vitamin D, magnesium, and zinc?"

If they're hesitant:

"Research shows these deficiencies can mimic or worsen mental health symptoms, especially in people who aren't responding fully to treatment."

Essential tests:

Ferritin (not just hemoglobin)	**B12**
Vitamin D	**Thyroid panel (TSH, Free T3, Free T4)**

If possible:

RBC magnesium	**Zinc**	**Copper (for zinc-copper ratio)**

3. Get actual numbers

Don't accept "everything's normal." Low-normal often isn't optimal:

> **What "normal" vs. "optimal" looks like:**
>
> **Ferritin:** "Normal" starts at 15, but many need above 50–75
>
> **Vitamin D:** "Normal" starts at 30, but 40–60 is often optimal
>
> **B12:** "Normal" starts at 200, but symptoms can occur below 400–500

4. Address deficiencies WITH your doctor

Important: Some supplements interact with psychiatric medications. Always discuss with your prescriber before starting anything.

Timelines:

Magnesium Days to weeks for some effects	**B12** Weeks to months
Iron 3–6 months to rebuild stores	**Vitamin D** 6–8 weeks

Continue your other treatment during this time. Minerals are one piece.

When Minerals Aren't the Answer

You've tested, supplemented, given it time. Still struggling.

Mental health condition needs different treatment: You might need different medication, higher dose, different therapy type, or more intensive treatment. Don't give up because minerals didn't fix everything.

Nervous system dysregulation is primary (Chapter 5): If you have significant trauma history, minerals can't override a dysregulated nervous system. Address nervous system work alongside or before expecting minerals to help.

Gut issues blocking absorption (Chapter 7): If you have digestive problems, you might not be absorbing supplements. Address gut health first.

Life circumstances: Sometimes depression and anxiety are responses to genuinely difficult situations. Minerals can't fix job loss, grief, or relationship problems. Therapy helps you cope, but sometimes circumstances need to change.

Protection—Safety—Healing Check-in

You just learned about brain function and minerals. Before you move on, notice where you are.

Struggling right now? This feels overwhelming?

That's okay. Here's the simple version: Keep your current treatment. Ask your doctor for one test: ferritin. That's it for now. If you're in crisis, call 988. You don't have to figure everything out today.

Stable but not thriving? Ready to investigate?

Good. Keep your current treatment. At your next appointment, request comprehensive testing—ferritin, B12, vitamin D, thyroid. Ask for actual numbers, not just "normal." Work with your doctor to address any deficiencies.

Doing okay? Want to optimize brain function?

Excellent. Request full testing including RBC magnesium and zinc. Consider whether nervous system work (Chapter 5) or gut healing (Chapter 7) might also support your mental health. Build comprehensive care that addresses biochemistry alongside therapy and lifestyle.

The Bottom Line

Your brain runs a neurotransmitter factory. Iron makes dopamine. Magnesium makes GABA. Zinc makes serotonin. When raw materials run low, the factory can't produce what you need—and medication alone can't compensate for missing building blocks.

Before they call it "treatment-resistant," get comprehensive testing: ferritin, B12, vitamin D, zinc, magnesium, thyroid.

But minerals are not a treatment for mental illness. They're one piece of comprehensive care that includes professional treatment, nervous system regulation, adequate sleep, and addressing life circumstances.

✔ **What to do:**

1. Continue your current treatment
2. Request comprehensive testing
3. Address deficiencies with your doctor's guidance
4. Give it time while continuing other treatment

✘ **What NOT to do:**

Stop medication to "try supplements instead"

Skip therapy because you think minerals are the answer

Delay getting help for a crisis

If you're struggling, please reach out. Talk to your doctor. See a therapist. Call 988 if you're in crisis.

You don't have to figure this out alone.

Crisis Resources

- 988 Suicide and Crisis Lifeline (24/7)
- Text HOME to 741741 Crisis Text Line
- 911 For immediate danger

Coming up in Chapter 12: Your heart beats 100,000 times a day without you thinking about it. But what happens when blood pressure creeps up? When your heart races for no reason? The next chapter tackles heart health—why magnesium matters for blood pressure and rhythm, how potassium protects your heart, and how to work with your doctor to protect the organ that keeps you alive.

CHAPTER 12

Heart and Blood Pressure

When your cardiovascular system struggles

You're at the doctor for a routine checkup. The nurse wraps the cuff around your arm, watches the numbers. Her eyebrows go up. She takes it again. Same result.

"Your blood pressure is a little elevated. The doctor will talk to you about it."

You're 45. Or 55. You eat pretty well. You exercise sometimes. How is your blood pressure high?

Or maybe it's not blood pressure. Maybe it's the flutter in your chest that wakes you at 3 AM. Your heart racing for no reason. A skipped-beat sensation that makes you catch your breath. You went to the cardiologist. They did an EKG. "Occasional PVCs," they said. "Benign. Nothing to worry about."

But it doesn't feel benign when your heart is doing somersaults.

So you talked to your doctor. For high blood pressure: "Cut back on salt." "Lose weight." "Here's a prescription." For the palpitations: "Reduce stress." "Cut caffeine." "Benign PVCs don't need treatment."

Maybe they prescribed medication. Maybe it helped. Maybe it caused side effects. Maybe you're on two or three medications now and your blood pressure still isn't quite controlled.

Here's what nobody told you: Your heart needs specific minerals to function properly. Every heartbeat requires a precise balance of magnesium, potassium, calcium, and sodium. When they're out of balance, blood pressure rises and heart rhythm becomes erratic.

They Said It Was Just Getting Older—They Were Wrong

"High blood pressure is just part of aging—take the medication and live with it."

TRUTH: Magnesium deficiency raises blood pressure. Magnesium relaxes blood vessel walls. When magnesium is low, vessels constrict and pressure goes up. Studies show magnesium supplementation lowers blood pressure by 3–4 mm Hg systolic—modest but clinically meaningful.

"Just cut back on salt and you'll be fine."

TRUTH: Potassium deficiency raises blood pressure. Potassium counterbalances sodium. The average American diet is extremely low in potassium and high in sodium—exactly wrong for blood pressure. Doctors say "cut back on salt" without addressing potassium. That's only half the equation.

"Benign PVCs don't need treatment—just ignore them."

TRUTH: Mineral imbalances cause heart rhythm problems. Your heart's electrical system depends on precise mineral balance. Low magnesium causes arrhythmias—including the "benign" PVCs that flutter in your chest. Yet most cardiologists don't check magnesium when patients complain of palpitations.

Your Heart Is a Muscle Too

Remember The Muscle Switch from Chapter 8? Calcium contracts muscles, magnesium relaxes them. When magnesium is low, your calf cramps at 2 AM because it's stuck in contraction.

Your heart is a muscle. Your blood vessels have smooth muscle in their walls. Same switch, same problem.

HEART MUSCLE

Each heartbeat = contract (calcium) then relax (magnesium). When magnesium is low, your heart can't relax fully between beats. Electrical signals become unstable. Result: palpitations, skipped beats, arrhythmias.

BLOOD VESSEL WALLS

Blood vessels need to relax to allow blood flow. When magnesium is low, vessel walls stay constricted. Result: higher pressure, harder work for your heart.

POTASSIUM = REGULATOR

Just like in skeletal muscle, potassium maintains proper electrical signaling. Low potassium → erratic signals → arrhythmias and blood pressure dysregulation.

The same switch that cramps your calf is squeezing your cardiovascular system all day long.

This is why magnesium is used intravenously in hospitals to treat certain dangerous arrhythmias. It works. Yet outpatient cardiologists rarely check it or recommend it for "benign" PVCs.

THE CRUEL IRONY

The most commonly prescribed blood pressure medications deplete the very minerals your heart needs.

Thiazide diuretics (hydrochlorothiazide, chlorthalidone):
Deplete potassium and magnesium.

Loop diuretics (furosemide/Lasix):
Deplete potassium, magnesium, and calcium.

You're prescribed medication that depletes minerals → which can raise blood pressure or cause arrhythmias → which requires more medication → which depletes more minerals.

"If you're on blood pressure medication and still not well-controlled, ask: Are my magnesium and potassium being monitored? Should I be supplementing to offset what the medication depletes?"

This single question has helped people break out of the escalating-medication cycle.

Your Kidneys Control Blood Pressure Too

Your kidneys aren't just filters. They're blood pressure regulators—controlling fluid balance, excreting or retaining sodium, and producing hormones that directly control BP.

Fluid Balance

Kidneys decide how much water to keep or release. More fluid = higher pressure.

Sodium Handling

Kidneys excrete excess sodium—but need potassium to do it properly.

Renin-Angiotensin System

Kidneys produce hormones that constrict blood vessels. Dysfunction = chronic vasoconstriction.

The Bidirectional Problem

High blood pressure damages kidneys. Kidney dysfunction raises blood pressure. They spiral together—which is why uncontrolled hypertension leads to kidney disease, and kidney disease worsens hypertension.

Minerals That Support Kidney Function

Magnesium: Helps kidneys excrete sodium properly. May help prevent kidney stones. Supports overall kidney function.

Potassium: Essential for the sodium-potassium pump—kidneys need potassium to get rid of excess sodium. Low potassium = sodium retention = higher BP.

Zinc and Selenium: Antioxidant properties may protect kidney tissue from damage.

The Balance Principle: It's Not Just "More"

Here's something critical to understand: your body needs mineral BALANCE, not maximum intake. Too little causes symptoms. Too much causes symptoms. The goal is optimal, not more.

Phosphorus: When More Becomes Dangerous

Unlike magnesium and potassium where deficiency is common, with phosphorus the problem is usually **excess**.

Where excess comes from: Processed foods (phosphate additives are everywhere), sodas (phosphoric acid), fast food

What excess phosphorus does: Pulls calcium from bones (bone disease), causes vascular calcification (hardening of arteries), arterial stiffness → higher blood pressure, strongly linked to cardiovascular disease

The kidney connection: Healthy kidneys excrete excess phosphorus. When kidney function declines, phosphorus builds up—and high phosphorus is a marker that kidneys aren't filtering properly.

⚠ THE CRITICAL FLIP

Here's what makes this complicated: once kidneys are impaired, this reverses.

Healthy kidneys benefit from adequate minerals. But damaged kidneys can't excrete excess minerals properly—so potassium and magnesium supplementation becomes dangerous, potentially fatal.

This is why kidney function must be checked before supplementing—especially potassium.

What to ask your doctor:

"Can we check my kidney function with a Cystatin C test along with my mineral levels? I understand it's more accurate than creatinine alone."

Why Cystatin C? Standard kidney tests (creatinine, eGFR) can be affected by muscle mass, diet, and hydration—and often don't show problems until significant damage has occurred. Cystatin C is produced by all cells at a constant rate, making it a more accurate and earlier indicator of kidney function.

Three Types of Cardiovascular Problems

1. High Blood Pressure

Readings consistently above 130/80. Often no symptoms—the "silent killer."

What's Happening: Blood vessels are constricted, creating resistance. This can be magnesium deficiency (vessels can't relax), potassium-sodium imbalance (fluid retention), arterial stiffness, kidney issues, sleep apnea, or chronic stress keeping you in fight-or-flight.

Mineral connections: Magnesium deficiency (vessel constriction), potassium deficiency (sodium retention, fluid imbalance), kidney dysfunction (renin-angiotensin dysregulation), sleep apnea (sympathetic activation).

What to discuss with your doctor:

"My blood pressure is elevated. Can we check magnesium and potassium before adding another medication?"

"Would the DASH diet be appropriate? I understand it works largely through increasing potassium and magnesium."

"Could I have sleep apnea? I understand it's a common cause of resistant hypertension."

If blood pressure isn't controlled on medication: Sleep apnea is one of the most common causes of resistant hypertension. Get a sleep study.

2. Palpitations and Arrhythmias

Racing heart, skipped beats, fluttering sensation, pounding heartbeat, irregular rhythm.

What's Happening: Your heart's electrical system is misfiring. Can be mineral imbalance (low magnesium, low potassium), stimulants, thyroid problems, anxiety, sleep apnea, or alcohol.

What to discuss with your doctor:

"I have palpitations and I understand these can be related to magnesium deficiency. Can we check my level? Even if it's 'normal,' could we try supplementation?"

"Is my potassium in the optimal range or just barely normal?"

"Has my thyroid been checked?"

What to track: Frequency of palpitations, triggers (caffeine, stress, alcohol, poor sleep), whether they change with magnesium supplementation.

Important:

If palpitations come with dizziness, fainting, chest pain, or severe shortness of breath—that needs urgent cardiac evaluation, not supplements.

3. Heart Failure

Shortness of breath with exertion, fatigue, leg swelling, reduced exercise capacity.

What's Happening: Your heart isn't pumping efficiently. Serious condition requiring medical management.

The mineral connection: Heart failure patients are often deficient in magnesium and potassium—from the condition itself and from diuretics used to treat it. Deficiencies worsen heart function and increase arrhythmia risk.

Heart failure is serious. Minerals are supportive, not a substitute for medical management. If you have heart failure symptoms, you need comprehensive cardiac evaluation.

Safety Check: When to Get Help Now

CALL 911 IMMEDIATELY:

- Chest pain or pressure with shortness of breath, sweating, or pain radiating to arm/jaw
- Severe sudden shortness of breath
- Fainting or loss of consciousness
- Blood pressure over 180/120 with symptoms (headache, chest pain, visual changes)
- Rapid heart rate (over 150) that won't slow down

SEE A DOCTOR THIS WEEK:

- Blood pressure consistently above 140/90
- New palpitations or change in pattern
- Chest discomfort with exertion
- New leg swelling

What minerals won't fix: Atrial fibrillation (requires medical management—blood thinners, rate control, possibly ablation), structural heart disease (valve problems, cardiomyopathy), coronary artery disease (blocked arteries need medical/surgical intervention), hypertensive emergency (needs immediate medical attention)

What Your Doctor Probably Doesn't Know

About magnesium and blood pressure: Meta-analyses confirm magnesium supplementation reduces blood pressure, particularly in deficient people. Yet magnesium is rarely checked in hypertension workup.

About magnesium and arrhythmias: Research clearly shows magnesium deficiency causes arrhythmias and supplementation reduces them. Yet cardiologists rarely check magnesium for "benign" PVCs.

About serum magnesium: It's unreliable—you can have "normal" serum magnesium while significantly deficient at the cellular level. RBC magnesium is more accurate but rarely ordered.

About the DASH diet: Proven to lower blood pressure as effectively as some medications. Works primarily by increasing potassium, magnesium, and calcium. Yet doctors often prescribe medication without first recommending dietary changes.

About sleep apnea: One of the most common causes of resistant hypertension. Dramatically under diagnosed. If your blood pressure isn't controlled on medication, get a sleep study.

Feel—Pause—Act: Before You Do Anything

If you're worried about your heart, pause before acting.

FEEL:

If you're on blood pressure medication, DO NOT stop taking it without your doctor's guidance. Stopping suddenly can cause dangerous rebound hypertension.

PAUSE:

Potassium supplementation can be dangerous if you have kidney disease or take certain medications (ACE inhibitors, ARBs). Too much potassium can cause fatal arrhythmias. Potassium supplements require medical guidance. Dietary potassium (fruits, vegetables) is generally safe.

ACT:

The goal is to optimize your cardiovascular care, not abandon it.

Calm action:
"I'll ask my doctor about checking magnesium and potassium at my next appointment while continuing my current treatment."

Working with Your Doctor

1. Continue current treatment

Keep taking medication. This chapter is about optimizing, not replacing.

2. Request testing

Say:

"I'd like to check whether mineral status might be contributing to my blood pressure/palpitations. Can we test magnesium and potassium?"

- Serum potassium (usually already checked)
- Serum magnesium (often NOT routinely checked—you need to ask)
- RBC magnesium if available (more accurate)

If you have resistant hypertension: Request a sleep study.

3. Interpret results carefully

Potassium: "Normal" is 3.5–5.0. Optimal for cardiovascular function is likely 4.0–5.0. If yours is 3.6, it's technically normal but may benefit from optimization.

Magnesium: "Normal" is 1.7–2.4. But serum is unreliable—you can be deficient with "normal" levels. If you're at the low end, deficiency is possible.

4. Discuss optimization

For magnesium:
"Can we try magnesium supplementation? Forms like glycinate or taurate are well-absorbed. What dose would you recommend?"

For potassium:
"Should I increase dietary potassium, or do I need supplements? Is supplementation safe given my medications and kidney function?"

If you're on diuretics:
"I know these can deplete minerals. Are my levels being monitored? Should I be supplementing?"

The DASH Diet Approach

8–14 mmHg

Blood pressure reduction in people with hypertension—comparable to medication

Why it works: Dramatically increases potassium (4,700 mg daily), magnesium, and calcium while moderating sodium.

The principles:

- Abundant vegetables and fruits (8–10 servings daily)
- Whole grains, lean protein, low-fat dairy
- Nuts and seeds
- Limited sodium (under 2,300 mg, ideally 1,500 mg)

This is mineral optimization through food. The mechanism is the same: more potassium and magnesium, better blood pressure.

What to ask:

"Would you support me trying the DASH diet for 8–12 weeks to see if it improves my blood pressure? Can we recheck then?"

When Minerals Aren't Enough

You've optimized minerals and diet. Blood pressure or rhythm problems persist.

You may need medication—and that's okay. Some people have cardiovascular issues requiring medication regardless of mineral status. Continue mineral optimization alongside medication.

Sleep apnea may be the cause. Extremely common, dramatically under diagnosed. If blood pressure isn't controlled, get a sleep study.

Structural heart problems: Valve issues, cardiomyopathy require cardiac evaluation and treatment.

Atrial fibrillation: Requires medical management—blood thinners, rate control, possibly ablation. Minerals support but don't cure AFib.

Nervous system dysregulation (Chapter 5): Chronic stress drives blood pressure up through elevated cortisol. If you're stuck in fight-or-flight, address that alongside minerals.

What to Track

Blood Pressure	Palpitations	Supplements
Check at same time daily, sit quietly 5 minutes first, track readings	Note when they occur, triggers, duration, associated symptoms	What you're taking, doses, any changes in blood pressure or symptoms

Bring this data to appointments.

Protection—Safety—Healing Check-in

You just learned about heart health and minerals. Before you move on, notice where you are.

Worried about your heart? This feels scary?

That's understandable. Here's the simple version: Keep taking your medication. Ask your doctor for one test: magnesium. That's it for now. If you have chest pain or severe symptoms, call 911.

Stable? Ready to optimize?

Good. Continue your current treatment. At your next appointment, request magnesium and potassium testing. Ask about DASH diet. If you snore or have uncontrolled blood pressure, discuss a sleep study.

Managing well? Want to reduce medication?

Excellent. Work with your doctor to try DASH diet for 8–12 weeks. Optimize minerals. Address stress (Chapter 5). Some people are able to reduce or eliminate blood pressure medication with lifestyle optimization—but only with medical supervision.

The Bottom Line

Your heart is a muscle. Your blood vessels have muscle walls. The Muscle Switch applies here too—calcium contracts, magnesium relaxes, potassium regulates.

When magnesium is low, your heart can't relax fully between beats (arrhythmias) and your blood vessels stay constricted (high blood pressure). The same switch that cramps your calf is squeezing your cardiovascular system.

The cruel irony: Common blood pressure medications deplete the very minerals your heart needs. If you're on diuretics, your magnesium and potassium should be monitored and likely supplemented.

The number to know: DASH diet can lower blood pressure 8–14 mm Hg—comparable to medication—primarily by increasing potassium and magnesium.

✔ What to do:

1. Continue current cardiovascular treatment
2. Request magnesium and potassium testing
3. If on diuretics, ask about supplementation
4. Consider DASH diet
5. If BP isn't controlled, get a sleep study
6. Address stress (Chapter 5)

✘ What NOT to do:

Stop blood pressure medication without guidance

Take potassium supplements without medical supervision

Ignore cardiovascular symptoms hoping minerals will fix them

Your heart beats 100,000 times a day. It deserves comprehensive care—medication when needed, minerals optimized, lifestyle supporting cardiovascular health.

Make the appointment. Ask for the testing. Have the conversation.

Coming up in Chapter 13: If you're a woman, your mineral needs change dramatically across your lifespan. Menstrual cycles, pregnancy, perimenopause, menopause—all shift what your body needs. The next chapter tackles hormonal health: why iron becomes critical during menstruating years, how magnesium helps PMS, what minerals support you through perimenopause and menopause, and how to work with your doctor when your hormones are shifting.

CHAPTER 13

Hormones: When Your Body Keeps Changing

Your body doesn't feel like your own anymore

You're lying in bed at 2 AM, drenched in sweat. Again. Third time this week. You were sound asleep and now you're wide awake, heart pounding, skin on fire.

Or maybe it's the week before your period when you turn into someone you don't recognize. Irritable. Weepy. Bloated. Your partner asks what's wrong and you want to scream—or cry—or both.

Or maybe you're so tired you can barely function, but your doctor says your thyroid is "fine." Your hair is falling out. You're gaining weight. You're freezing all the time. Nobody believes you.

Or maybe you're bleeding so heavily during your period that you're afraid to leave the house. You've ruined clothes, chairs, car seats. You're exhausted all the time. Your doctor offered birth control or suggested a hysterectomy. Nobody mentioned checking your iron.

So you went to your doctor. For the hot flashes: "Welcome to menopause. It's just something you have to get through." For the PMS: "That's normal. Some women just have it worse." For the thyroid symptoms: "Your TSH is normal. Maybe you're depressed." For the heavy periods: "Some women just bleed heavily. Here's birth control."

Here's what nobody told you: Your hormones and minerals are deeply interconnected. Magnesium helps regulate PMS. Iron depletion from heavy periods causes crushing fatigue that looks like depression. Zinc and selenium are required for thyroid hormone conversion. When doctors treat hormonal symptoms without checking mineral status, they're missing half the picture.

They Said It Was "Just Hormones"—They Were Partly Right

Yes, hormones are involved. But hormones don't exist in a vacuum. They require minerals to be produced, converted, and function properly.

"PMS is just something women have to deal with."

TRUTH: Magnesium deficiency makes PMS worse. Research shows women with PMS have lower magnesium levels. Studies demonstrate magnesium supplementation significantly reduces PMS symptoms—mood changes, bloating, breast tenderness, cramps. Yet doctors rarely check magnesium for PMS. They offer birth control or antidepressants.

"You're just depressed—here's an antidepressant."

TRUTH: Heavy periods cause iron deficiency that mimics depression. Women who bleed heavily lose significant iron every month. Low iron causes crushing fatigue, low motivation, brain fog, feeling emotionally flat—symptoms identical to depression. Women get diagnosed with depression and prescribed antidepressants when the real problem is iron deficiency.

"Your TSH is normal, so your thyroid is fine."

TRUTH: Thyroid function requires minerals. Your thyroid needs iodine to make hormones, selenium to convert T4 to T3 (active form), zinc for conversion and receptor function, and iron for production. You can have "normal" TSH but still feel terrible if minerals are preventing proper hormone function.

Your Endocrine System Is a Factory

Like the neurotransmitter factory in Chapter 11, your endocrine system produces hormones. Minerals are the raw materials.

THYROID HORMONES

Iodine + Selenium + Zinc

→ T4 → T3 (active hormone)

Without iodine, no hormone gets made.

Without selenium and zinc, T4 can't convert to T3.

STRESS HORMONES

Magnesium regulates cortisol. When magnesium is low, cortisol stays elevated.

This affects every other hormone—thyroid, reproductive, everything.

REPRODUCTIVE HORMONES

Iron enables production. Magnesium helps regulate the cycle.
B vitamins support metabolism.

Heavy periods deplete iron, worsening the cycle.

When raw materials run low, the factory malfunctions. You get symptoms—but labs might look "normal" because standard tests don't check the raw materials.

THE DEPRESSION THAT ISN'T DEPRESSION

If you have heavy periods AND crushing fatigue, low motivation, brain fog, and flat mood—and your doctor diagnosed depression:

Ask for your ferritin level.

Women with heavy periods can lose several times more iron per cycle than those with lighter periods. Over months and years, this depletes iron stores even if hemoglobin stays "normal."

Low ferritin causes symptoms identical to depression:

• Crushing fatigue • No motivation • Can't concentrate • Feeling emotionally flat • Brain fog

Women get prescribed antidepressants when they need iron.

The Number

Ferritin above 50

Many women with ongoing blood loss need 75–100 to feel normal

If your ferritin is below 50 and you bleed heavily, you likely have your answer. This single test has changed lives for women who spent years on antidepressants for a problem that was never depression.

WHEN "NORMAL" THYROID ISN'T NORMAL

If you have thyroid symptoms—fatigue, weight gain, cold intolerance, brain fog, hair loss, constipation—and your doctor said "your thyroid is fine" based on TSH:

Ask for Free T3.

Your thyroid makes mostly T4 (inactive). It must convert to T3 (active) to work. This conversion requires selenium and zinc.

You can have "normal" TSH and T4 but low T3—because conversion isn't happening. Your labs look fine. You feel terrible.

Also ask about: Selenium, zinc, and thyroid antibodies (TPO, thyroglobulin). Hashimoto's thyroiditis is autoimmune—your immune system attacks your thyroid. Selenium supplementation reduces antibodies and may slow the disease.

If Free T3 is low-normal and you have symptoms, mineral deficiency might be the missing piece. Correcting selenium and zinc can improve thyroid function—sometimes dramatically—without medication.

Four Hormonal Situations

1. Severe PMS or PMDD

Mood changes, irritability, anxiety, crying spells, bloating, breast tenderness in the week before your period. Symptoms resolve when period starts. PMDD is the severe, disabling form.

What's Happening: Your brain is sensitive to normal hormonal fluctuations. Magnesium levels drop during the luteal phase, worsening symptoms.

What to discuss with your doctor:

"Research shows magnesium 200–400 mg daily reduces PMS symptoms. Can I try this?"

"Should I also try calcium (1,000–1,200 mg daily)? Studies show it helps PMS too."

"Would B6 supplementation be appropriate?"

Timeline: Give it 2–3 cycles to assess.

If minerals alone aren't enough: PMDD is severe and requires going back to Part II. Your nervous system regulation (Chapter 5) directly affects hormonal balance. Your signaling pathways (Chapter 6) determine whether hormones communicate properly. Your gut health (Chapter 7) affects estrogen metabolism. Address all three systems alongside minerals. Additional support may include vitex (chasteberry), omega-3s, blood sugar stability, and possibly bioidentical progesterone. If your symptoms are truly disabling—not just difficult, but disabling—SSRIs have strong research support and are worth discussing with your doctor. For most cyclical symptoms that don't reach that level, minerals address the underlying biology first.

2. Heavy Periods and Fatigue

Periods lasting more than 7 days, soaking through protection every 1–2 hours, passing large clots, limiting activities due to flow. Crushing fatigue, especially around your period.

What's Happening: You're losing significant iron every month. Over time, ferritin depletes even if hemoglobin stays "normal."

What to discuss with your doctor:

"I have heavy periods and I'm exhausted. Can we check ferritin, not just hemoglobin?"

"If ferritin is low, what iron supplementation do you recommend?"

"What's causing my heavy bleeding? Do I need a pelvic ultrasound?"

Important:

Iron supplementation replaces what you're losing, but doesn't stop the bleeding. The underlying cause (fibroids, adenomyosis, hormonal imbalance) needs treatment too—hormonal IUD, medication, or other intervention.

Timeline: You may feel somewhat better within weeks, but rebuilding stores takes 3–6 months.

3. Thyroid Symptoms with "Normal" Labs

Fatigue, weight gain, feeling cold, constipation, dry skin, hair loss, brain fog, depression. Or the opposite (hyperthyroid): racing heart, weight loss, anxiety, feeling hot, tremor.

What's Happening: If you have hypothyroid symptoms but "normal" TSH, possibilities include:

- TSH is "normal" but at the high end (3–4.5) where many people feel terrible
- T4 isn't converting to T3 due to selenium or zinc deficiency
- Autoimmune thyroid (Hashimoto's)—positive antibodies but normal TSH early in disease

What to discuss with your doctor:

"My TSH is [number] but I have symptoms. Can we check Free T3, Free T4, and thyroid antibodies?"

"Can we check selenium and zinc? They're required for T4 to T3 conversion."

"If I have Hashimoto's, research shows selenium 200 mcg daily reduces antibodies. Would this be appropriate?"

If your doctor dismisses symptoms with "normal" TSH, consider a second opinion from an endocrinologist or integrative medicine doctor.

Warning:

Hyperthyroid symptoms (racing heart, tremor, weight loss, anxiety) need medical evaluation. Hyperthyroidism is dangerous—don't self-treat.

4. Perimenopause and Menopause

Irregular periods, hot flashes, night sweats, sleep disturbances, mood changes, brain fog, vaginal dryness. After 12 months without a period, you're in menopause.

What's Happening: Ovaries producing less estrogen and progesterone. This is natural, but symptoms can be severe.

The honest truth about minerals and menopause:

Hot flashes: Minerals don't dramatically help. Hormone therapy is most effective. Don't suffer for years when effective treatment exists.

Sleep and mood: Magnesium can help.

Bone protection: This is where minerals become critical.

After menopause, without estrogen's protection, bone loss accelerates. You need:

- Calcium: 1,000–1,200 mg daily
- Vitamin D: enough to maintain blood level 40–60 ng/mL
- Magnesium: 300–400 mg daily
- Vitamin K2: 100–200 mcg daily (directs calcium to bones)

What to discuss with your doctor:

"My symptoms are affecting my quality of life. Can we discuss hormone therapy? What are the actual risks and benefits for me?"

"For bone protection, can we check my vitamin D? What supplementation do you recommend?"

"Should I get a DEXA scan for baseline bone density?"

About hormone therapy: The risks have been overstated. For most women under 60 or within 10 years of menopause, HRT is safe and dramatically improves quality of life. Don't suffer because you're afraid of it.

Safety Check: When to Get Help Now

SEE A DOCTOR THIS WEEK:

- Bleeding so heavy you're soaking through protection every hour
- Any bleeding after menopause (needs evaluation to rule out cancer)
- Severe pelvic pain
- Symptoms of severe anemia (extreme fatigue, shortness of breath, racing heart)
- Rapid heart rate, severe anxiety, tremor (hyperthyroidism can be dangerous)

WHAT MINERALS WON'T FIX:

- PMDD (requires comprehensive holistic approach; for severe PMDD, SSRIs are well-supported by research and often first-line)
- Fibroids/polyps (need gynecological treatment)
- Hyperthyroidism (needs medical treatment)
- Severe hypothyroidism (may need medication)
- Severe osteoporosis (may need medication beyond minerals)

What Your Doctor Probably Doesn't Know

About PMS: Magnesium supplementation reduces PMS symptoms in multiple studies. Yet gynecologists rarely recommend it.

About heavy periods and iron: Ferritin should be checked in any woman with heavy periods and fatigue—not just hemoglobin. A ferritin of 20 is "normal" but often symptomatic with ongoing blood loss.

About thyroid: Selenium is essential for T4-to-T3 conversion. Selenium supplementation improves thyroid function and reduces antibodies in Hashimoto's. Yet endocrinologists rarely check selenium or recommend it.

About "normal" TSH: The range (0.5–4.5) is statistically derived, not based on how people feel. Many people have symptoms with TSH of 3–4. Optimal is often 1–2.

About menopause and HRT: The risks were overstated. For most women, benefits outweigh risks. Many suffer needlessly because they're afraid of hormone therapy.

Feel—Pause—Act: Before You Do Anything

If you've been dismissed for years, you may be desperate for answers. Pause.

FEEL:

If you're on thyroid medication, keep taking it. If you're on hormone therapy, keep taking it. Minerals are added to treatment, not replacements.

PAUSE:

Don't stop any current treatment while investigating mineral status.

ACT:

One step. One conversation.

Calm action:

"I'll ask my doctor to check ferritin at my next appointment" or "I'll discuss magnesium for PMS" or "I'll ask for Free T3, not just TSH."

Working with Your Doctor

For PMS:
"Research shows magnesium reduces PMS symptoms. Can we check my level and discuss supplementation?"

For heavy periods:
"I have heavy periods and fatigue. Can we check ferritin specifically? And what's causing my heavy bleeding?"

For thyroid:
"I have symptoms but my TSH is normal. Can we check Free T3, Free T4, and antibodies? And selenium and zinc status?"

For menopause:
"Can we discuss hormone therapy? I also want to make sure I'm protecting my bones—can we check vitamin D?"

Key tests to request:

Ferritin (for heavy periods/fatigue)	**Free T3, Free T4, thyroid antibodies**
Magnesium, vitamin D, B12	**Selenium, zinc** (if thyroid symptoms)

When Minerals Aren't Enough

For PMS/PMDD: Go back to Part II—nervous system regulation (Chapter 5), signaling (Chapter 6), gut health (Chapter 7). Add vitex, omega-3s, blood sugar stability. Work with a holistic practitioner. For severe PMDD, SSRIs have strong research support and may be appropriate alongside these approaches.

For heavy periods: The bleeding itself needs treatment—hormonal IUD, medication, ablation, or addressing fibroids. Don't just supplement iron forever.

For thyroid: If you genuinely have hypothyroidism, you need medication. Minerals support but don't replace thyroid hormone when it's needed.

For menopause: Hormone therapy is the most effective treatment for severe symptoms. Minerals support but won't eliminate hot flashes.

Protection—Safety—Healing Check-in

You just learned about hormones and minerals. Before you move on, notice where you are.

Exhausted and overwhelmed? Been dismissed for years?

That's understandable. Here's the simple version: If you have heavy periods + fatigue, ask for ferritin. If you have thyroid symptoms + "normal" TSH, ask for Free T3. One test. That's your starting point.

Managing symptoms? Ready to investigate?

Good. Identify which situation matches yours (1–4). Request the specific tests for your situation. Continue current treatments while investigating. Track symptoms across 2–3 cycles if hormonal.

Stable? Want to optimize hormonal health?

Excellent. Get comprehensive mineral testing. Address gut health (Chapter 7) for estrogen metabolism. Balance nervous system (Chapter 5) for cortisol regulation. Consider working with an integrative practitioner for holistic hormonal support.

The Bottom Line

Your endocrine system is a factory. Hormones are the products. Minerals are the raw materials.

Iodine + selenium + zinc → thyroid hormones. Magnesium → regulates stress response and PMS. Iron → enables production (and is depleted by heavy periods).

When raw materials run low, the factory malfunctions. You get symptoms—but standard tests often miss the problem.

The depression that isn't depression: Heavy periods + fatigue + low mood often equals iron deficiency, not depression. Ask for ferritin.

The "normal" thyroid that isn't normal: Symptoms with normal TSH may mean poor T4-to-T3 conversion. Ask for Free T3 and mineral status.

✓ What to do:

1. Continue current hormonal treatments
2. Request mineral testing based on your symptoms
3. Address deficiencies found
4. If minerals aren't enough, pursue appropriate medical treatment

✗ What NOT to do:

Stop thyroid medication to try supplements

Avoid hormone therapy out of fear when you might benefit

Ignore severe symptoms hoping minerals will fix everything

Stop antidepressants to try iron supplements as a fourth bullet, parallel to the thyroid medication line

Your hormones change throughout your life. Minerals support you through all transitions—but they work best as part of comprehensive care.

Make the appointment. Ask for the testing. Have the conversation.

Coming up in Chapter 14: You wash your hands, you try to sleep enough—and you still catch every cold that goes around. The next chapter tackles immunity: why zinc is the commander of your immune response, how selenium protects against viral infections, and how to work with your doctor when you're getting sick too often.

CHAPTER 14

Immunity: When You Catch Everything

You're always sick

It's February and you're on your third cold of the winter. Or maybe your fourth—you've lost count. You just got over the last one when the next one hit.

Your coworkers come to work sick, cough on everything, and recover in three days. You catch whatever they have and you're down for two weeks. Every time.

Or maybe it's not colds. Maybe it's the sinus infection that won't clear. The bronchitis that lingers for a month. The stomach bug that flattens you while everyone else recovers in 24 hours. The cut that takes forever to heal.

You wash your hands. You try to sleep. You take vitamin C when you feel something coming on. Nothing helps.

Your doctor said: "Some people just catch more colds." "Your immune system is probably fine." "Try to get more rest."

Here's what nobody told you: Your immune system is an army. And your army is starving.

The Army Framework

Think of your immune system as a military force defending your body. Like any army, it needs resources to function:

ZINC
=
THE COMMANDER

Develops, activates, and coordinates your immune cells. Without adequate zinc, your T-cells can't mature, your natural killer cells can't attack, your antibodies can't form. The commander is missing, and the troops don't know what to do.

SELENIUM
=
THE ARMOR

When immune cells fight pathogens, they generate reactive oxygen species—cellular weapons. Without selenium, your own immune cells get destroyed in the crossfire. Selenium-dependent antioxidants protect your troops from burning out in battle.

VITAMIN D
=
THE INTELLIGENCE

Activates antimicrobial defenses and coordinates the response. It tells your immune system when to attack and—critically—when to stand down. Without intelligence, your army either doesn't show up or overreacts.

IRON
=
THE SUPPLY LINE

Rapidly dividing immune cells need iron. When you mount an immune response, cell numbers expand dramatically. Iron delivers oxygen to immune tissues and supports this rapid deployment.

When these resources run low, your army can't defend you. You catch everything. You stay sick forever. Infections that others fight off in days take you down for weeks.

Standard blood work doesn't check this. So you keep getting sick while the real problem goes unaddressed.

WHY "COLD AND FLU SEASON" EXISTS

It's not the cold weather. It's not being indoors together.

It's vitamin D.

During winter months in northern latitudes, your skin can't make vitamin D from sun—even on sunny days. The angle is wrong. Vitamin D levels plummet across the population. Respiratory tract defenses weaken. Everyone catches everything.

"Cold and flu season" is largely vitamin D deficiency season.

The Number

Vitamin D above 40 ng/mL

For optimal immune function. Most people in winter are below 30. Many are below 20.

If you live above the 37th parallel (San Francisco to Richmond, Virginia, to Athens, Greece), you likely can't make vitamin D from November through February. Supplementation isn't optional—it's required.

Three Patterns of Poor Immunity

1. You Catch Everything

Multiple colds per year. Every stomach bug hits you. Kids bring home illness and you always get it.

What's Happening: Your surveillance and first-line defenses aren't working. Pathogens that others' immune systems catch early are getting a foothold in you.

The mineral connection: Zinc deficiency impairs barrier function and first-response. Vitamin D deficiency weakens respiratory defenses. Check both.

2. You Stay Sick Forever

When you get sick, you're down for weeks. Colds turn into sinus infections. Cuts heal slowly. You feel wiped out long after the acute illness resolves.

What's Happening: Your immune system can't mount an effective response, or your troops are burning out in the process of fighting.

The mineral connection: Zinc is essential for tissue repair. Selenium protects immune cells from oxidative damage. Iron deficiency means tissues aren't getting oxygen for recovery. All three need investigation.

3. The Same Infection Keeps Returning

Cold sores that keep coming back. Recurrent UTIs. Chronic sinus infections. Multiple courses of antibiotics for the same problem.

What's Happening: Your immune system can't fully eliminate pathogens, or barriers in a specific area are compromised.

The mineral connection: Zinc is critical for barrier integrity. But recurrent specific infections often need medical investigation beyond minerals—structural issues, blood sugar problems, or conditions requiring specific treatment.

Don't assume it's "just minerals." Recurrent infections in the same location warrant proper medical evaluation.

Safety Check

THIS WEEK if you have:

- Fever over 103°F or lasting more than 3 days
- Signs of serious infection (severe pain, confusion, difficulty breathing)
- Infection that's rapidly worsening
- Severe wound infection (spreading redness, red streaks, pus)

SOON if you have:

- More than 4–6 respiratory infections per year
- Infections that always require antibiotics
- Pneumonia more than once
- Infections that don't respond to standard treatment
- Unexplained weight loss with frequent infections

WHAT MINERALS WON'T FIX:

- Primary immunodeficiency (rare genetic conditions)
- HIV/AIDS or other secondary immunodeficiency
- Immunosuppression from medications or chronic disease
- Autoimmune conditions
- Chronic infections requiring specific treatment

Red flag: If you're getting unusual infections—organisms that don't typically cause disease in healthy people—that's a sign of significant immune dysfunction requiring thorough evaluation.

The Selenium Secret

Here's something most doctors don't know: Selenium deficiency doesn't just weaken your response to viruses—it makes viruses more dangerous.

Research demonstrated that normally mild strains of influenza and coxsackievirus became more virulent when they replicated in selenium-deficient hosts. The virus itself mutated into a more dangerous form.

Your selenium status doesn't just affect whether you get sick. It affects how dangerous the virus becomes inside you.

Selenium is rarely checked. Deficiency is common in many geographic areas because soil selenium varies dramatically. Parts of the Pacific Northwest and East Coast have low soil selenium—food grown there contains less.

One to two Brazil nuts daily provides adequate selenium for most people. It's that simple.

Feel—Pause—Act

FEEL

If you're currently sick: This isn't the time to start multiple new supplements. Rest, hydrate, recover. Zinc lozenges within 24 hours of cold onset may help shorten duration, but don't overhaul your regimen while fighting infection.

PAUSE

If you're between illnesses: This is when to optimize. But address systematically, not desperately.

ACT

Calm action:
"I'll ask my doctor to check zinc, vitamin D, and selenium"—not "I'll order every immune supplement tonight."

Working with Your Doctor

Say this:

"I've been getting sick frequently—[describe your pattern]. I'd like to check whether mineral deficiency might be contributing. Can we test zinc, vitamin D, and selenium?"

Tests to request:

Serum zinc (normal 60–120 mcg/dL; low-normal may still be suboptimal)

25-hydroxy vitamin D (below 30 is insufficient; aim for 40–60)

Selenium (normal 70–150 ng/mL)

Ferritin if you also have fatigue

If deficient:

ZINC

15–30 mg daily. Don't exceed 40 mg long-term without monitoring—high zinc depletes copper.

VITAMIN D

1,000–5,000 IU daily depending on deficiency severity. Retest in 2–3 months.

SELENIUM

100–200 mcg daily, or 1–2 Brazil nuts. Don't exceed 400 mcg—selenium toxicity is real.

Building Your Defenses

Food first:

ZINC

Oysters (highest by far), beef, crab, chicken dark meat, pumpkin seeds, chickpeas.

SELENIUM

Brazil nuts (1–2 daily is enough), fish, eggs, meat.

VITAMIN D

Sunlight (10–30 min midday), fatty fish, egg yolks. Supplements often necessary.

Part II matters here too:

Gut health (Chapter 7): Your gut houses 70–80% of your immune system. You can't have good immunity without good gut health.

Sleep (Chapter 9): Sleep deprivation dramatically impairs immune function. People sleeping less than 7 hours are significantly more likely to catch colds.

Stress (Chapter 5): Chronic stress suppresses immunity through elevated cortisol. Nervous system regulation directly supports immune function.

Exercise: Moderate exercise enhances immunity. Extreme exercise temporarily suppresses it—the "open window" after hard workouts when athletes get sick.

During cold/flu season:

If you live in northern latitudes: Vitamin D3 supplementation (1,000–2,000 IU daily) is reasonable for most adults even without testing.

Zinc lozenges at cold onset: Research shows zinc lozenges (13–23 mg zinc acetate or gluconate, dissolved in mouth every 2–3 hours) started within 24 hours can reduce cold duration by 1–3 days.

What about vitamin C? You probably already reach for it—everyone does. It does support immune function and may modestly help at illness onset. But vitamin C isn't the forgotten nutrient. Zinc, selenium, and vitamin D are—and for the person who catches everything, they may matter more.

When Minerals Aren't Enough

You've optimized zinc, vitamin D, and selenium. You've addressed sleep, stress, and gut health. You're still getting sick constantly.

Consider:

Other nutritional factors: Protein deficiency impairs antibody production

Chronic conditions: Uncontrolled diabetes significantly impairs immunity

Underlying immune dysfunction: Some people have primary immunodeficiencies diagnosed in adulthood—if unusual or severe infections persist, immunology referral is appropriate

Lifestyle factors: Smoking dramatically impairs respiratory immunity. Heavy alcohol suppresses immune function. No supplement overcomes these.

What Success Looks Like

You won't become immune to everything. The goal:

- Fewer infections per year (2–3 colds instead of 6+)
- Faster recovery (days instead of weeks)
- Less severe symptoms
- Fewer complications (colds staying colds, not becoming bronchitis)

Timeline: Building immune resilience takes months. If you optimize in summer, assess over the following winter. One illness isn't the measure—patterns over a season are.

Protection—Safety—Healing Check-in

You just learned about immunity and minerals. Before you move on, notice where you are.

Currently sick? Just getting over something?

That's okay. Focus on recovery first. Rest, hydrate. Zinc lozenges if within 24 hours of symptoms. Save the testing and optimization for when you're well.

Between illnesses? Ready to build defenses?

Good. Request testing for zinc, vitamin D, and selenium. Start vitamin D if you're in northern latitudes. Add 1–2 Brazil nuts daily. Address sleep and stress from Part II.

Generally healthy? Want to optimize?

Excellent. Get baseline testing. Optimize through food first—oysters, Brazil nuts, fatty fish. Address gut health (Chapter 7). Build the complete system so when cold season hits, your army is ready.

The Bottom Line

Your immune system is an army that needs resources to defend you. Zinc commands the response. Selenium protects your troops from burning out. Vitamin D provides intelligence. Iron supports rapid deployment.

When these run low—which is common—you catch everything and stay sick forever.

"Cold and flu season" is really vitamin D deficiency season.

The person who catches every bug often has zinc deficiency.

The one whose infections drag on forever may be burning through selenium.

Give your army what it needs. Stop being the person who catches everything.

Next: You push your body—at the gym, on trails, in competition. But when you're depleted, performance suffers and recovery stalls. Chapter 15 tackles exercise and athletic performance.

CHAPTER 15

Exercise and Athletic Performance

When your body can't keep up

You're three miles into a run you've done a hundred times. Your legs feel like concrete. Your lungs are burning. Your heart is pounding way harder than it should be. You used to cruise through this route. Now you're wondering if you can make it home.

Or maybe it's the weights that used to feel manageable now feeling impossibly heavy. The bike ride that leaves you wrecked for two days. The gym session where you bonk halfway through and can't figure out why.

You're not that old. You're not that out of shape. Something is wrong.

Or maybe it's not during the workout—it's after. You're destroyed for days. Muscle soreness that won't quit. Feeling worse, not better, from the activity that's supposed to make you healthy.

Your doctor said: "You're probably overtraining." "Take some rest days." "Maybe you're just getting older."

Here's what nobody told you: Your body is a performance machine. And your machine is missing critical parts.

The Performance Machine

Think of your body like a high-performance engine. It needs specific components to function:

IRON = FUEL DELIVERY

Iron carries oxygen from your lungs to your working muscles. No iron, no oxygen delivery. Your muscles suffocate while you gasp for air that can't get where it needs to go.

MAGNESIUM = THE BATTERY

Every muscle contraction runs on your body's energy currency. But that energy only works when magnesium is attached. Without enough magnesium, your muscles can't access the power they need. The battery is dead.

ELECTROLYTES = ELECTRICAL SYSTEM

Your muscles run on electrical signals. Sodium, potassium, calcium, and magnesium create those signals—telling muscles when to fire and when to relax. When electrolytes get depleted, the wiring shorts out.

Remember The Muscle Switch from Chapter 8? Calcium contracts, magnesium relaxes, potassium regulates. That same switch controls every movement you make during exercise—thousands of times per workout.

When these components run low, your performance machine sputters. And here's the problem: exercise depletes all of them.

You lose iron through pounding impact (which destroys red blood cells in your feet), through tiny amounts of gut bleeding during intense exercise, and through sweat. You lose magnesium in sweat and because hard training uses more of it. You lose electrolytes with every drop of sweat. The harder you train, the more you deplete.

THE TEST YOUR SPORTS PHYSICAL DOESN'T INCLUDE

If your performance is declining and you've been told "your iron is fine," ask:

What was my ferritin?

Standard sports physicals check hemoglobin—that's the iron in your blood right now. If it's normal, case closed. But ferritin—your iron stores—can be 15, 20, 25 while hemoglobin stays normal. You're not anemic. You're just running on fumes.

Research clearly shows: Iron deficiency WITHOUT anemia impairs athletic performance. Your heart pounds harder at normal paces. You fatigue faster. Your endurance tanks. Your times get slower.

The Number for Athletes

Ferritin above 35–50

Many sports medicine experts recommend even higher for endurance athletes. Female athletes—who lose iron monthly on top of exercise losses—are at highest risk.

Your sports physical said you're fine. Your ferritin says otherwise.

Three Patterns of Exercise Problems

1. Declining Performance Despite Training

Your times are getting slower. Workouts feel harder at the same intensity. You can't hit paces or power numbers you used to. Heart rate is higher than expected for the effort.

What's Happening: Your machine can't deliver or use fuel efficiently.

The mineral connection: Iron deficiency reduces oxygen delivery—even without anemia. Magnesium deficiency impairs energy production. Both are common in athletes and rarely checked.

2. Poor Recovery and Prolonged Soreness

Muscle soreness that lasts 4–5 days instead of 1–2. Feeling wrecked after workouts that used to be routine. Needing more rest days than before. Fatigue that accumulates week over week.

What's Happening: Your body can't repair damage and adapt efficiently.

The mineral connection: Magnesium and zinc are essential for protein synthesis—muscle repair. Magnesium deficiency also impairs sleep (Chapter 9), which is when recovery actually happens. Iron deficiency means tissues don't get oxygen for repair.

3. Cramping and Muscle Issues

Cramps during or after exercise. Night cramps after hard training days. Muscle twitches, spasms, tightness that won't release.

What's Happening: The electrical system is malfunctioning.

The mineral connection: Magnesium deficiency is the most common cause—magnesium is required for muscle relaxation. Sodium depletion from heavy sweating. Potassium depletion. Often multiple electrolytes are depleted simultaneously.

Safety Check

STOP EXERCISING AND GET HELP IMMEDIATELY if:

- Chest pain or pressure
- Severe shortness of breath
- Dizziness or fainting
- Irregular heartbeat that doesn't resolve with rest
- Dark brown or red urine after exercise (this means muscle is breaking down—it's a medical emergency)

THIS WEEK if:

- Persistent fatigue that doesn't improve with rest
- Performance decline that doesn't respond to program changes
- Signs of iron deficiency (extreme fatigue, pale skin, racing heart)
- Heart palpitations during or after exercise

WHAT MINERALS WON'T FIX:

- True overtraining syndrome (requires extended rest—weeks to months)
- Not eating enough to support your training (you need more food, not more supplements)
- Heart conditions causing exercise symptoms
- Eating disorders (common in athletes; requires treatment beyond supplementation)

If you're restricting food, over-exercising, or have lost your period (females), please address this. No supplement fixes undereating.

The Sweat Tax

Every time you exercise, you pay a mineral tax in sweat. The longer and harder you go, the more you pay.

Average losses per liter of sweat:

Sodium: 800 mg (ranges 460–1,840)

Potassium: ~200 mg

Magnesium: 10–25 mg

Zinc: 0.5–1 mg

If you sweat 2 liters during a workout—common in endurance exercise or heat—you might lose 1000+ mg sodium, 400+ mg potassium, and meaningful amounts of magnesium and zinc.

Over weeks and months of training, these losses compound. Some athletes are "salty sweaters"—you can see salt crusts on skin or clothing. These athletes are at even higher risk.

You're depleting faster than you realize. And "eating well" doesn't automatically replace what you're losing.

Feel—Pause—Act

FEEL

If you're mid-training-cycle: Don't make dramatic changes before important events. Competition week isn't for experimenting.

PAUSE

If your body is screaming for rest: Listen. Minerals support recovery but don't replace it.

ACT

Calm action:

"I'll ask my doctor to check ferritin before next season"—not "I'll start iron without testing." Never supplement iron without knowing your levels. Too much is harmful.

Working with Your Doctor

Say this:

"I'm training [hours per week]. I want to check whether mineral status is affecting my performance. Can we test ferritin—not just hemoglobin?"

Tests to request:

Complete blood count (includes hemoglobin)	**Ferritin** (your iron stores—critical)
Vitamin D	**Magnesium**

Understanding your results:

Ferritin: Lab "normal" starts at 15. That's not good enough for athletes. Target 35–50 or higher. Below 20? That's likely dragging down your performance.

Vitamin D: Below 30 is too low. 40–60 is the sweet spot for performance and bone health.

If ferritin is low:

- Work with your doctor on dose (typically 30–65 mg daily)
- Ask for iron bisglycinate—it's a gentler form that's easier on your stomach
- Take with vitamin C to help absorption
- Don't take with coffee, tea, or calcium (they block absorption)
- Retest in 8–12 weeks

Caution: Don't supplement iron without testing. Some people have a condition that causes iron overload—they should never take iron supplements. Always test first.

If magnesium is low or you're cramping:

- 300–400 mg daily (look for magnesium glycinate or citrate—they absorb well)
- Take at night (helps sleep)
- Generally safe—your body gets rid of any extra

Fueling the Machine

Iron Sources

Red meat (your body absorbs this best), poultry dark meat, fish, shellfish, beans, fortified cereals. If eating plant sources, have them with vitamin C to help absorption.

Magnesium Sources

Pumpkin seeds, almonds, spinach, black beans, dark chocolate, avocado.

Electrolyte replacement during exercise:

For workouts over 60 minutes or any exercise in heat:

- Replace sodium (sports drinks, salt tablets, salted foods)
- Don't just drink plain water during long/hot events—you need electrolytes
- Practice your fueling strategy in training, not race day

For shorter workouts in moderate conditions: Water is usually sufficient if your overall diet is good.

Part II matters here too:

Sleep (Chapter 9) is when recovery happens. No supplement overcomes chronic sleep deprivation.

Rest days are not optional. Your body adapts during recovery, not during the workout.

Stress management (Chapter 5) affects recovery capacity. Training stress + life stress = total stress load.

Special Considerations

Female athletes: Higher risk for iron deficiency because you lose iron monthly on top of exercise losses. Get your ferritin checked regularly—at least once or twice a year. If your period is irregular or has stopped, that's a medical issue that needs attention.

Endurance athletes: You sweat more, which means greater losses. You also destroy more red blood cells through impact and have higher iron turnover. Get ferritin checked regularly. Pay close attention to replacing electrolytes during long training sessions and races.

Plant-based athletes: Iron and zinc from plants are harder for your body to absorb. You may need supplements even with a "good" diet. B12 supplements are required—there are no plant sources. Plant-based eating can absolutely support excellent performance, but you need to pay more attention to these nutrients.

Athletes over 40: Mineral optimization becomes more important with age, not less. Don't accept "you're just getting older" without investigation.

When Minerals Aren't Enough

You've addressed mineral status. You're eating enough. You're sleeping. You're still struggling.

Consider:

True overtraining syndrome: Your body is broken down and needs extended rest (weeks to months), not supplements

Not eating enough: If you're not fueling your training, no supplement will fix it—you need more food

Medical conditions: Thyroid problems, lingering viral infections, heart conditions, autoimmune disease

Training program issues: Too much volume, not enough recovery, poor planning

Life stress: If you're maxed out in life, your body has less capacity for training stress

Sometimes the answer is training less, not supplementing more.

What Success Looks Like

Addressing deficiencies takes time:

IRON	MAGNESIUM	VITAMIN D
2–3 months to rebuild stores.	Some effects in days-weeks (cramping, sleep), full benefits take longer.	2–3 months to reach optimal levels.

You won't go from struggling to setting personal records overnight. But you should see:

- Training feeling more manageable at the same intensity
- Heart rate appropriate for effort level
- Recovering normally between sessions
- Cramping resolved or dramatically reduced
- Sleeping better
- Feeling like yourself again

Protection—Safety—Healing Check-in

You just learned about exercise and minerals. Before you move on, notice where you are.

Performance tanking? Exhausted from training?

That's a signal. Get ferritin tested—not just hemoglobin. Consider taking a rest week while you investigate. Your body is telling you something.

Training okay but not thriving? Ready to optimize?

Good. Request baseline testing: ferritin, vitamin D, magnesium. Address what you find. Pay attention to electrolyte replacement during long sessions. Build recovery into your program.

Performing well? Want to prevent problems?

Excellent. Get annual ferritin testing, especially if female or endurance athlete. Optimize recovery through sleep and nutrition. Consider your total stress load—training + life. Prevention is easier than recovery.

The Bottom Line

Your body is a performance machine that needs specific components to function. Iron delivers fuel. Magnesium powers the battery. Electrolytes run the electrical system.

Exercise depletes all of them. The harder you train, the more you lose. "Sports anemia" is real. The ferritin test your sports physical doesn't include is often the answer.

Don't accept "you're just overtraining" or "you're just getting older" without investigation.

Get ferritin tested—not just hemoglobin. Address what you find. Replace what you're losing.

Your body is capable of remarkable things. Give it the components it needs, and it can do what you're asking of it.

Next: Your hair is thinning. Your nails are brittle. Your skin looks dull. These aren't just cosmetic concerns—they're visible signals from your body that something is wrong inside. Chapter 16 tackles the external signs of internal deficiency.

CHAPTER 16

Hair, Skin, and Nails

When your body shows you something is wrong

You're brushing your hair and the brush is full again. Not a few strands—clumps. You find hair on your pillow, in the shower drain, on your clothes. Your ponytail is half the thickness it used to be.

Or maybe it's your nails—so brittle they peel and break before they grow past your fingertips. Ridges running down them like tiny mountain ranges. Nails that split and crack no matter what you do.

Or maybe it's your skin. Dry patches that won't go away no matter how much moisturizer you use. A small cut that takes weeks to heal instead of days. Skin that just doesn't look healthy anymore.

Your dermatologist said: "It's probably stress." "It's genetic." "Have you tried Rogaine?" "Some women just lose hair after 40." For the nails: "Use nail strengthener." "Keep them moisturized." For the skin: "Here's a cream." "Try a different moisturizer."

Maybe you've spent hundreds of dollars on hair treatments, nail products, and expensive skincare. Nothing really fixes the problem.

Here's what nobody told you: Your body runs a triage system. And your hair, skin, and nails are last in line.

The Triage System

When resources are scarce, your body makes hard choices. It's like an emergency room during a disaster—the most critical patients get treated first.

FIRST PRIORITY

Heart, brain, and liver are critical. They get minerals first. Always.

LAST IN LINE

Hair, skin, and nails aren't essential for survival. They get what's left over.

This means something important: When your hair, skin, and nails start changing, your body is so depleted it can't even maintain your exterior. These tissues are your body's early warning system. They show deficiency before anything else does—precisely because they're last in line for resources.

That hair falling out isn't just a cosmetic problem. It's your body saying: **"I'm so low on iron that I can't spare any for hair follicles."**

Those brittle nails aren't just annoying. They're your body saying: **"I don't have enough zinc to build strong proteins."**

That dry, slow-healing skin isn't just aging. It's your body saying: **"I'm running on empty."**

These visible changes are messages. And the message is: something is wrong inside.

WHY YOUR DERMATOLOGIST DIDN'T CHECK YOUR IRON

If you're losing hair and your dermatologist recommended Rogaine without checking your ferritin: **Go back and ask.**

Research shows women with unexplained hair loss have significantly lower ferritin than women without hair loss. Iron deficiency—even without anemia—causes hair loss. Your hair follicles are among the fastest-dividing cells in your body. They need constant iron-rich blood supply to function.

The Number for Hair Health

Ferritin above 70

Not 15 (where "normal" starts). Not 30. Above 70.

Dermatologists focus on topical treatments. They're not trained to think of hair loss as a sign of internal deficiency. So women spend years trying products to fix hair loss that's caused by low iron. Your body is telling you something. Your dermatologist may not have been listening.

What These Tissues Need

Hair

Hair is made of protein (keratin). Your hair follicles are tiny factories that produce keratin and push it up as a hair shaft. These factories need:

Iron: Delivers oxygen to the follicle. Without it, follicles can't keep up with rapid cell division.

Zinc: Required for making protein. Deficiency weakens hair and disrupts the growth cycle.

Thyroid hormones: Control the whole operation. Both underactive and overactive thyroid cause hair loss.

Skin

Skin is your largest organ—a protective barrier that completely replaces itself every 4–6 weeks. That constant renewal requires:

Zinc: Essential for cell division, wound healing, and controlling oil production.

Iron: Delivers oxygen for repair.

Vitamin C: Required for collagen (the protein that gives skin structure).

Nails

Nails grow from a matrix at the base of the nail bed. They grow slowly—about 3mm per month—so nail changes reflect what was happening in your body weeks to months ago.

Iron: Severe deficiency causes spoon-shaped nails (edges curve upward).

Zinc: Needed for protein production. Deficiency causes slow growth and brittleness.

Biotin: Involved in keratin production. Has actual research support for improving brittle nails.

Four Patterns

1. Hair Loss (Diffuse Thinning)

Hair coming out in clumps. Overall thinning rather than bald patches. Ponytail thinner than before. Maybe thinning eyebrows, especially the outer third.

What's Happening: When something stresses your body—illness, surgery, crash dieting, severe stress, or nutritional deficiency—hair follicles go into "rest mode." Two to four months later, those hairs fall out. This is why hair loss often appears months AFTER whatever caused it.

The mineral connection: Iron deficiency is the most common nutritional cause in women. Zinc deficiency also causes hair loss. Thyroid problems (both under and overactive) cause diffuse thinning.

2. Skin Problems

Chronically dry skin despite moisturizing. Slow wound healing. Acne that doesn't respond to topical treatment. Cracks at the corners of your mouth.

What's Happening: Your skin can't renew itself properly without the right building blocks.

The mineral connection: Zinc is the key mineral for skin. It's involved in cell division, wound healing, and oil regulation. Zinc deficiency causes dry skin, slow healing, acne, and those cracks at the mouth corners. Iron deficiency causes pale, dry skin.

3. Brittle Nails

Nails break or peel easily. Won't grow past fingertips. Splitting, ridges, slow growth.

What's Happening: Your nail matrix can't produce strong keratin without the right materials.

The mineral connection: Iron deficiency causes brittle nails (severe deficiency causes spoon-shaped nails). Zinc deficiency causes slow growth and brittleness. Biotin supplementation has research support for improving nail strength.

4. Everything at Once

Hair loss AND brittle nails AND skin problems—all happening together.

What's Happening: When multiple tissues are affected, it's a sign of significant systemic deficiency.

The mineral connection: Iron and zinc deficiency both affect all three. Thyroid problems affect all three. This pattern needs thorough investigation, not just topical treatment.

When everything is affected at once, that's a signal to investigate internally—not to buy more products.

Safety Check

THIS WEEK if:

- Sudden, rapid hair loss (losing clumps daily)
- Signs of skin infection (spreading redness, warmth, pus, fever)
- New rash with fever or feeling unwell

SOON if:

- Significant hair loss lasting more than a few weeks
- Patchy hair loss (bald patches)—this could be an autoimmune condition
- Persistent skin changes that don't respond to basic care
- Any hair/skin/nail changes with other symptoms (fatigue, weight changes, mood changes)

WHAT MINERALS WON'T FIX:

- Genetic pattern hair loss (may need medication or other treatments)
- Autoimmune hair loss (alopecia areata—patchy bald spots)
- Autoimmune skin conditions (psoriasis, lupus)
- Fungal infections (need antifungal treatment)
- Skin cancer (any new or changing mole needs evaluation)

Feel—Pause—Act

Changes in your appearance can feel urgent. You want to fix it now.

But hair loss took months to develop—hairs that shifted to "rest mode" 2–4 months ago are just now falling out. Regrowth will also take months. **There's no overnight fix.**

Calm action:
"I'll ask my doctor to check ferritin, zinc, vitamin D, and thyroid before trying products"—not "I'll buy every hair supplement on Amazon."

And don't take iron without testing first. Too much iron is harmful. Always test before supplementing.

Working with Your Doctor

Say this:

"I'm experiencing [hair loss/skin changes/brittle nails]. I'd like to check whether nutritional deficiency might be contributing before trying topical treatments. Can we test ferritin, zinc, vitamin D, and thyroid?"

Tests to request:

Complete blood count (checks for anemia)

Ferritin (iron stores—this is the key test for hair loss)

TSH (thyroid screening)

Vitamin D

Zinc

Understanding your results:

Ferritin: Lab "normal" starts at 15. For hair health, aim for 70 or higher. If you have hair loss and ferritin below 50, iron deficiency is a likely contributor.

Thyroid (TSH): Above 4.0–4.5 suggests underactive thyroid. Below 0.5 suggests overactive. Both cause hair, skin, and nail changes.

Vitamin D: Below 30 is too low. Deficiency is linked to hair loss.

If ferritin is low:

- Work with your doctor on dose
- Ask for iron bisglycinate (gentler on your stomach)
- Take with vitamin C to help absorption
- Don't take with coffee, tea, or calcium (they block absorption)
- Hair regrowth takes 6–12 months after iron comes back up—be patient

If zinc is low:

- 15–30 mg daily
- Take with food
- Don't exceed 40 mg daily long-term

About biotin: It has actual research support for brittle nails (2.5–5 mg daily). But tell your doctor if you're taking it—high-dose biotin can interfere with some lab tests, including thyroid tests.

Building Healthy Tissues

Protein matters: Hair, skin, and nails are made of protein. If you're not eating enough, your body can't build these tissues.

Iron Sources	Zinc Sources	Biotin Sources
Red meat (your body absorbs this best), poultry, fish, beans, fortified cereals. Pair plant sources with vitamin C.	Oysters (highest), beef, crab, chicken, beans, nuts, seeds.	Eggs (cooked—raw egg whites actually block biotin absorption), nuts, salmon, avocado.

Part II matters here too: Sleep (Chapter 9), stress management (Chapter 5), and gut health (Chapter 7) all affect hair, skin, and nails. A body under chronic stress doesn't have resources to spare for your exterior.

Special Situations

Postpartum hair loss: Extremely common 2–4 months after childbirth. During pregnancy, hormones kept hair in growth mode. After delivery, all those hairs that didn't fall out during pregnancy fall out at once. Usually resolves by 6–12 months, but iron deficiency (from blood loss during delivery) can contribute. Worth checking ferritin.

After crash dieting or weight loss: Severe calorie restriction causes hair loss 2–4 months later. Your body shunted resources to vital organs. You may need to eat more. Hair will recover once nutrition is restored, but it takes time.

Menopause: Hormone changes can cause hair thinning, dry skin, and nail changes. Mineral optimization supports your body during this transition.

What Success Looks Like

These tissues recover slowly. Set realistic expectations:

Hair

- Loss slows in 2–4 months
- New growth in 3–6 months
- Significant improvement: 6–12 months
- Full regrowth: 12–18 months

Skin

- Wound healing improves in weeks
- Skin texture improves in 1–3 months

Nails

- Fingernails grow ~3mm/month
- Improvement visible: 3–6 months
- Full replacement: 6 months

Take photos at the start and monthly. Changes are gradual and hard to notice day-to-day.

Protection—Safety—Healing Check-in

You just learned about hair, skin, nails and minerals. Before you move on, notice where you are.

Hair falling out in clumps? Distressed by changes?

That's understandable—these changes are visible and upsetting. Get ferritin and thyroid tested before trying products. One test may give you the answer. And remember: regrowth takes months, so patience is part of the process.

Noticing changes? Ready to investigate?

Good. Request comprehensive testing: ferritin, zinc, vitamin D, thyroid. Identify which pattern matches your symptoms. Address what you find. Take photos to track progress.

Tissues healthy? Want to keep them that way?

Excellent. Ensure adequate protein, iron, and zinc in your diet. Address sleep and stress (Part II). Consider annual ferritin testing, especially if female or vegetarian. Prevention is easier than regrowth.

The Bottom Line

Your hair, skin, and nails are last in line for resources. **When they start changing, your body is telling you it's so depleted it can't maintain your exterior.**

These aren't cosmetic problems to cover up with products. They're signals to investigate.

Iron deficiency causes hair loss—even without anemia.

Zinc deficiency affects skin, hair, and nails.

Thyroid problems show up in all three.

Get tested before you treat. Ask for ferritin, zinc, vitamin D, and thyroid. Address what you find. Be patient—these tissues recover in months, not days.

Your body is sending you visible signals. Don't just cover them up. Understand them.

→ ***Next:* *Part IV*** *brings it all together—how to troubleshoot when things aren't working, how to maintain optimal status long-term, and how to build habits that actually stick.*

PART IV

Making It Work

You've learned what minerals do.
You've identified what might be blocking you.
You've connected symptoms to possible deficiencies.

Now comes the part most books skip: what to do when it Doesn't go smoothly.

In This Section:

CHAPTER 17

Troubleshooting

When things don't go as planned

Permission to Quit

Before we troubleshoot: You're allowed to stop.

If a supplement makes you feel worse, stop taking it. If the process is causing more stress than your symptoms, take a break. If you've tried everything and nothing helps, minerals might not be your answer—and that's okay. You have permission to close this book and revisit later, or not at all.

Things Will Go Wrong

This isn't pessimism. It's realism.

You'll take a supplement that gives you diarrhea. You'll get labs that don't make sense. You'll feel worse before you feel better. You'll forget to take things for weeks. You'll wonder if any of this is working.

This is normal. This is part of the process. This doesn't mean you're failing.

Feel—Pause—Act: When Problems Arise

FEEL

Notice what's actually happening—in your body AND in your nervous system. Are you frustrated? Panicking? Disappointed?

PAUSE

Don't throw out all your supplements. Don't spiral into "nothing works." Don't give up entirely. Just pause.

ACT

From a calmer place, make one small adjustment. Not a complete overhaul—one change at a time.

Quick Reference

Problem	**Try This First**	**#**
Magnesium → diarrhea	Switch to glycinate form, lower dose	**1**
Iron → constipation/nausea	Take with food, try gentle form	**2**
Any supplement → side effects	Lower dose, different form, take with food	**3**
Labs normal but still symptomatic	Check optimal vs. normal ranges	**4**
3 months, no improvement	Check absorption blockers, retest	**5**
Can't afford supplements/tests	Food first, prioritize one test	**6**
Doctor won't order tests	Use script language, or direct-to-consumer	**7**
Can't stay consistent	Lower the bar, 4–5 days is enough	**8**

1. "I took magnesium and now I have diarrhea"

What's happening:

Magnesium draws water into your intestines. Some forms (especially oxide and citrate) do this more than others. This is actually how Milk of Magnesia works as a laxative.

Try this:

Switch forms. Magnesium glycinate is gentler on digestion. Lower your dose and build up slowly. Split doses throughout the day instead of taking all at once.

When to worry: If diarrhea is severe, bloody, or lasts more than a few days after stopping, see your doctor.

2. "Iron makes me constipated/nauseous"

What's happening:

Iron is hard on the digestive system. This is one of the most common reasons people stop taking it—even when they desperately need it.

Try this:

Take with food (even though absorption is slightly lower). Try a gentler form like iron bisglycinate. Start with a lower dose and increase gradually. Take every other day instead of daily—research shows this can actually improve absorption while reducing side effects.

When to worry: Black, tarry stools (not just dark from iron) or severe abdominal pain need medical attention.

3. "I'm having side effects from [any supplement]"

General troubleshooting:

1. **Lower the dose**—try half or even quarter dose
2. **Try a different form**—same mineral, different compound
3. **Take with food**—even if label says empty stomach
4. **Try a different brand**—fillers and additives vary
5. **Stop and reassess**—some bodies just don't tolerate certain supplements

4. "My labs are normal but I still feel terrible"

What's happening:

"Normal" lab ranges are designed to catch disease, not identify optimal function. You can be technically "normal" and still functionally deficient.

Check these:

Ferritin: "Normal" starts at 12–15. Optimal is above 50–70.

Vitamin D: "Normal" starts at 30. Many feel better at 50–70.

B12: "Normal" starts around 200. Symptoms can occur below 500.

Trust your body. "Normal" doesn't mean optimal. If you feel terrible, keep investigating.

5. "I've been supplementing for 3 months with no improvement"

Check these potential blockers:

Are you actually absorbing? Low stomach acid, gut issues, and certain medications can block absorption even with adequate intake.

Are you taking the right form? Some forms are poorly absorbed (magnesium oxide, zinc oxide).

Is the dose adequate? Some supplements are underdosed—check if you're actually getting therapeutic amounts.

Is something else going on? Chronic inflammation, thyroid issues, or other conditions can cause similar symptoms.

> **Next step:** Retest. If levels haven't improved despite supplementation, you have an absorption problem—revisit Part II.

6. "I can't afford supplements or testing"

Prioritize ruthlessly:

One test: If you can only afford one test, make it ferritin (for women) or vitamin D (for everyone). These are the most commonly deficient and most likely to cause symptoms.

Food first: Prioritize mineral-rich foods before supplements. Canned sardines, pumpkin seeds, dark leafy greens, and eggs give you a lot of minerals for little money.

Generic is fine: Store-brand supplements are often identical to expensive brands. Check the ingredient list.

Direct-to-consumer labs: Companies like Ulta Labs and Walk-In Lab offer testing without a doctor's order, sometimes cheaper than copays.

7. "My doctor won't order the tests I want"

Try this language:

> **Say this:**
>
> "I'm experiencing [specific symptoms]. I'd like to rule out mineral deficiency as a contributing factor. Can we check ferritin, vitamin D, and magnesium RBC?"

If they still refuse: Ask them to document the refusal in your chart. This often changes minds. If not, consider direct-to-consumer testing or finding a different provider.

8. "I can't stay consistent"

Reframe this:

Perfect consistency is not the goal. 4–5 days per week is enough for most supplements. You're not failing if you miss days.

FEEL

"I'm frustrated that I keep forgetting."

PAUSE

"This is just a story. Lots of people struggle with consistency. Missing days doesn't erase progress."

ACT

"I'll put them next to my coffee maker and aim for weekdays only."

When to Get Medical Help

Call 911 or go to the ER if:

Chest pain, difficulty breathing, severe allergic reaction, confusion, or fainting after taking any supplement.

Call your doctor same day if:

Severe digestive distress, rash or hives, heart palpitations, or significant worsening of symptoms.

Schedule an appointment if:

Mild but persistent side effects, no improvement after 3 months, or confusing lab results.

The Bottom Line

Problems are information, not failure. Adjust, adapt, or move on. Your body will tell you what it needs—keep listening.

→ *Continue to Chapter 18: Long-Term Maintenance*

CHAPTER 18

Long-Term Maintenance

Keeping what you've gained

What Maintenance Actually Looks Like

Here's what most people think maintenance looks like: You fix your deficiencies. You feel better. You keep doing exactly what you did to get there. Forever. With perfect consistency.

Here's what it actually looks like:

You feel better for a while. Then you get busy and forget supplements for two weeks. Then you restart. Then you feel fine and wonder if you still need them. Then you stop. Then three months later symptoms return. Then you restart.

Messy. Imperfect. Non-linear. Human.

FEEL: Notice when symptoms start returning.

PAUSE: Don't spiral into "everything's broken again."

ACT: Adjust based on what your body needs right now.

That's it. Stay attuned to your body. Make small adjustments as needed. Live your life.

Your Maintenance Cheat Sheet

Mineral	Treatment Dose	Maintenance Dose	Retest
Iron	25–65 mg daily	Often none; 30–65 mg EOD if needed	Every 6–12 mo
Magnesium	400–600 mg daily	200–300 mg daily or 400 mg 3–4x/wk	Every 1–2 yr
Zinc	30–40 mg daily	15–30 mg daily	Annually
Vitamin D3	4,000–10,000 IU daily	1,000–2,000 IU daily	Every 1–2 yr

Vitamin D3 doses above 4,000 IU should be guided by blood levels and supervised—toxicity is possible with prolonged high doses.

Warning signs to restart supplementing:

- Muscle cramps or tension returning → magnesium
- Fatigue, hair loss, heavy periods → check ferritin
- Low mood in winter → vitamin D
- Slow wound healing, frequent illness → zinc
- Sleep disruption after a calm period → magnesium

You can skip testing when:

- You're taking low doses within RDA ranges
- You feel consistently well
- You can't afford it and you're managing fine by feel

When to Stop vs. Stay on

"I've been taking magnesium for six months and feel great. Do I need it forever?"

Answer: Maybe. Try stopping and find out.

Symptoms return in days/weeks? → You need it. Restart. This is your maintenance dose.

Symptoms return after months? → Supplement seasonally or restart when symptoms appear.

Symptoms don't return? → You fixed it. Stay off unless things change.

To test: Choose a calm time. Stop one supplement at a time. Give it 4–6 weeks. Track the specific symptoms that supplement addressed.

Some supplements correct a deficiency—you might not need them forever. Others compensate for ongoing needs—you might need them indefinitely. There's no shame in long-term supplementation. That's just your body's reality.

The 80/20 Rule

20% that gives 80% of results

- ✔ Pay attention to your body's signals
- ✔ Address deficiencies that clearly affect your life
- ✔ Maintain food sources
- ✔ Retest every 1–2 years if supplementing long-term

80% that only gives 20%

- ✘ Perfect timing (morning vs. evening rarely matters)
- ✘ Perfect daily consistency (4–5 days/week is enough)
- ✘ Taking every mineral "just in case"
- ✘ Obsessive tracking or constant testing

Focus on what matters. Be okay with "good enough" on everything else.

The Maintenance Mantra

Regulated First, Optimized Second

When you're regulated, you hear your body's signals clearly. You troubleshoot without panicking. You can be flexible. You stop things that aren't serving you.

When you're dysregulated, every symptom feels like crisis. You can't tell if something's working. You feel like you're always failing.

The most important maintenance practice is staying regulated enough to listen to your body and respond appropriately.

Sometimes the best maintenance decision is to stop trying to maintain and just live your life.

If tracking minerals creates more anxiety than your symptoms did, stop. You can always come back.

> You don't owe anyone—including yourself—perfect optimization.
>
> **You owe yourself a life that feels good to live.**

→ ***Continue to the Conclusion***

CONCLUSION

Your Next Steps

What This Book Was Really About

Let me tell you what this book wasn't about.

It wasn't about turning you into a minerals expert. It wasn't about giving you one more thing to optimize, track, or feel bad about. And it definitely wasn't about convincing you that if you just get your magnesium perfect, all your problems will disappear.

This book was about three things:

First, giving you permission to trust your body again.

The medical system has spent your whole life teaching you not to trust your body's signals. You're tired? Push through. You're in pain? It's probably stress. Your labs are fine, so nothing's wrong with you.

This book said: What if your body is telling you the truth? What if that exhaustion isn't a character flaw but iron deficiency? What if those cramps aren't something to tolerate but a sign you need magnesium?

Second, making decisions from regulation instead of desperation.

When you feel terrible and nothing works, you make decisions from panic. Buy everything. Try seventeen things at once. Swing between obsessive optimization and complete avoidance.

Feel-Pause-Act gave you a different way. Notice what's happening. Calm your nervous system. Then make one small, informed adjustment.

Third, taking action without needing it to be perfect.

You don't have to implement everything. You just have to try one thing. See what happens. Adjust. Try again.

That's success—engaging with your health from curiosity and self-compassion instead of shame and fear.

The Three Core Truths

If you remember nothing else:

1. Your symptoms are real, even when your labs are "normal."

Standard lab ranges catch disease, not suboptimal function. You can have ferritin of 15 (normal) and feel exhausted. Trust your body's signals. Keep investigating.

2. Food first, supplements second—but supplements aren't cheating.

The best way to get minerals is from whole foods. But if you're deficient, supplements can be genuinely helpful and sometimes necessary. You're not failing if you need to supplement.

3. Regulated first, optimized second. Always.

If tracking minerals makes you anxious, if you feel controlled by your supplement routine, if every symptom sends you into panic—you're not optimizing health. You're dysregulating your nervous system. Sometimes the healthiest thing is to stop trying to optimize and just live your life.

The One Action to Take This Week

Not five actions. **One.**

1. Request one specific test from your doctor based on your symptoms.
2. Try one supplement for one symptom. Take it consistently for 4 weeks. See what happens.
3. Increase one food source for two weeks.
4. Stop one thing that isn't serving you.
5. Do nothing differently—just pay attention to your body for a week.

Pick one. Do it this week. That's enough.

How to Know If Minerals Are Helping

Minerals ARE helping if:

✔ Specific symptoms improve

✔ The improvement lasts

✔ When you stop, symptoms return

✔ Lab values improve

Minerals are NOT helping if:

✗ Nothing changes after 3–4 months

✗ Symptoms get worse

✗ Labs don't improve despite supplementation

✗ You can't tolerate any form

Be honest about what's happening. Give things a fair trial. Assess honestly. Adjust or move on.

When to Move on

It's time to move on from minerals when:

- You've addressed deficiencies and feel better (shift to maintenance)
- You've given it a fair trial with no improvement (minerals probably aren't your answer)
- The pursuit of optimization is making you more anxious than the symptoms did
- You have bigger priorities right now

If minerals weren't your answer, other places to look:

Sleep quality • Chronic stress • Hormonal imbalances • Blood sugar • Gut issues • Autoimmune conditions • Mental health • Environmental toxins • Social isolation • Lack of purpose

Health has many factors. Minerals are one piece. If they're not your piece, that's okay.

The Last Thing

I'm going to tell you something I wish someone had told me years ago:

You are not broken. You never were.

Your body was telling you the truth. The problem was that the systems designed to help you couldn't hear what your body was saying. Or wouldn't listen. Or didn't have the tools.

But you're learning to hear it now. You're learning to trust yourself again.

You don't need to be perfect at this. You don't need to track fourteen minerals and achieve optimal levels and maintain flawless consistency forever.

You just need to pay attention. Make small adjustments when needed. Respond with curiosity and compassion instead of shame and fear.

That's it. That's the practice.

Permission to Close This Book

Put it down.

Don't add it to your growing list of health projects you "should" finish. Don't feel guilty that you didn't implement every suggestion.

Just do one thing. This week. One small thing that might help you feel a little better.

Your body was telling you the truth. Now you're learning to listen.

And that—that skill, that practice, that trust—is worth more than all the magnesium in the world.

You don't need to be perfect.

You just need to start.

And you already have.

APPENDIX A—SOURCES AND REFERENCES

This appendix provides peer-reviewed scientific sources organized by the themes and chapters in this book. References include systematic reviews, meta-analyses, and landmark studies supporting the evidence-based concepts presented. All citations include DOI where available.

PART I: MINERAL ESSENTIALS

Magnesium Fundamentals and Distribution

1. Jahnen-Dechent W, Ketteler M. Magnesium basics. Clinical Kidney Journal. 2012;5(Suppl 1):i3-i14. doi:10.1093/ndtplus/sfr163. Serum magnesium represents only 0.3% of total body magnesium; ~99% is stored in bone, soft tissue, and muscle.

2. de Baaij JH, Hoenderop JG, Bindels RJ. Magnesium in man: implications for health and disease. Physiological Reviews. 2015;95(1):1–46. doi:10.1152/physrev.00012.2014. Comprehensive review of magnesium homeostasis and clinical implications.

Iron Deficiency and Anemia

3. Camaschella C. Iron-deficiency anemia. New England Journal of Medicine. 2015;372(19):1832–1843. doi:10.1056/NEJMra1401038. Iron deficiency can occur without anemia; evidence on pre-anemia symptoms varies. [Note: Extent of nonhematologic effects before anemia remains unclear.]

4. Lopez A, Cacoub P, Macdougall IC, Peyrin-Biroulet L. Iron deficiency anaemia. The Lancet. 2016;387(10021):907–916. doi:10.1016/S0140-6736(15)60865-0. Comprehensive review of iron deficiency diagnosis and management.

5. Allen RP, Picchietti DL, Auerbach M, et al. Evidence-based and consensus clinical practice guidelines for the iron treatment of restless legs syndrome. Sleep Medicine. 2018;41:27–44. doi:10.1016/j.sleep.2017.11.1126. Guidelines recommend iron supplementation when ferritin is ≤75 μg/L in RLS patients.

Laboratory Testing and Assessment

6. Arnaud MJ. Update on the assessment of magnesium status. British Journal of Nutrition. 2008;99(Suppl 3):S24-S36. doi:10.1017/S000711450800682X. Critical review of magnesium testing methods; serum Mg has limited sensitivity for detecting deficiency.

7. Lowe NM, Fekete K, Decsi T. Methods of assessment of zinc status in humans: a systematic review. American Journal of Clinical Nutrition. 2009;89(6):2040S-2051S. doi:10.3945/ajcn.2009.27230G. Systematic review comparing different methods for assessing zinc status.

Mineral Forms, Bioavailability, and Supplementation

8. Schuette SA, Lashner BA, Janghorbani M. Bioavailability of magnesium diglycinate vs magnesium oxide in patients with ileal resection. JPEN. 1994;18(5):430–435. doi:10.1177/0148607194018005430. In malabsorption patients, diglycinate showed higher absorption in poorest absorbers (23.5% vs 11.8%). [Note: Subgroup finding, not general population.]

9. Firoz M, Graber M. Bioavailability of US commercial magnesium preparations. Magnesium Research. 2001;14(4):257–262. Magnesium oxide has ~4% fractional absorption vs higher rates for chloride, lactate, aspartate.

10. Stoffel NU, Cercamondi CI, Brittenham G, et al. Iron absorption from oral iron supplements given on consecutive versus alternate days. The Lancet Haematology. 2017;4(11):e524-e533. doi:10.1016/S2352-3026(17)30182-5. Alternate-day dosing achieves 40–50% higher fractional iron absorption due to hepcidin dynamics.

11. Moretti D, Goede JS, Zeder C, et al. Oral iron supplements increase hepcidin and decrease iron absorption from daily or twice-daily doses. Blood. 2015;126(17):1981–1989. doi:10.1182/blood-2015-05-642223. Mechanistic study explaining hepcidin increase lasting ~24 hours after iron dosing.

12. Gómez-Ramírez S, Brilli E, Tarantino G, Muñoz M. Sucrosomial iron: a new generation iron for improving oral supplementation. Pharmaceuticals. 2018;11(4):97. doi:10.3390/ph11040097. Review of sucrosomial iron technology showing improved tolerability and absorption characteristics compared to conventional iron salts.

Drug-Nutrient Interactions

13. U.S. Food and Drug Administration. FDA Drug Safety Communication: Low magnesium levels can be associated with long-term use of PPIs. FDA Safety Communication. March 2, 2011. PPIs used >1 year may cause hypomagnesemia requiring supplementation or discontinuation.

14. Heidelbaugh JJ. Proton pump inhibitors and risk of vitamin and mineral deficiency. Therapeutic Advances in Drug Safety. 2013;4(3):125–133. doi:10.1177/2042098613482484. Review of PPI effects on B12, magnesium, calcium, and iron absorption.

PART II: UNDERSTANDING YOUR BODY

Nervous System, Stress, and Mineral Depletion

15. Seelig MS. Consequences of magnesium deficiency on the enhancement of stress reactions. Journal of the American College of Nutrition. 1994;13(5):429–446. doi:10.1080/07315724.1994.10718432. Landmark paper on how stress depletes magnesium and deficiency amplifies stress responses.

16. Pickering G, Mazur A, Trousselard M, et al. Magnesium status and stress: the vicious circle concept revisited. Nutrients. 2020;12(12):3672. doi:10.3390/nu12123672. Review of bidirectional relationship between magnesium deficiency and stress.

17. Takase B, Akima T, Uehata A, et al. Effect of chronic stress and sleep deprivation on intracellular magnesium level. Clinical Cardiology. 2004;27(4):223–227. doi:10.1002/clc.4960270411. Stress and sleep deprivation reduce intracellular magnesium levels.

18. Sartori SB, Whittle N, Hetzenauer A, Singewald N. Magnesium deficiency induces anxiety and HPA axis dysregulation. Neuropharmacology. 2012;62(1):304–312. doi:10.1016/j.neuropharm.2011.07.027. Magnesium deficiency upregulates the HPA axis, increasing ACTH and CRH.

Peptide and Hormonal Signaling

[Principle-level references. For the mineral-specific application, see refs 2 and 77 for magnesium and refs 10 and 11 for hepcidin's control of iron.]

19. Kohan DE, Inscho EW, Wesson D, Pollock DM. Physiology of endothelin and the kidney. Compr Physiol. 2011;1(2):883–919. doi:10.1002/cphy.c100039. PMID: 23737206.

20. Russo D, Pisani A, Balletta MM, De Nicola L, Savino FA, Andreucci M, Minutolo R. Additive antiproteinuric effect of converting enzyme inhibitor and losartan in normotensive patients with IgA nephropathy. Am J Kidney Dis. 1999;33(5):851–6. doi:10.1016/s0272-6386(99)70416-6. PMID: 10213639.

21. Krishnamurthy P, Rajasingh J, Lambers E, Qin G, Losordo DW, Kishore R. IL-10 inhibits inflammation and attenuates left ventricular remodeling after myocardial infarction via activation of STAT3 and suppression of HuR. Circ Res. 2009;104(2):e9–18. doi: 10.1161/CIRCRESAHA.108.188243. PMID: 19096025.

22. Bocalini DS, Carvalho EV, de Sousa AF, Levy RF, Tucci PJ. Exercise training-induced enhancement in myocardial mechanics is lost after 2 weeks of detraining in rats. Eur J Appl Physiol. 2010;109(5):909–14. doi: 10.1007/s00421–010–1406-x. PMID: 20300769.

23. Zhang H, Dellsperger KC, Zhang C. The link between metabolic abnormalities and endothelial dysfunction in type 2 diabetes: an update. Basic Res Cardiol. 2012;107(1):237. doi:10.1007/s00395-011-0237-1. PMID: 22189563.

24. Andersson C, Vasan RS. Epidemiology of heart failure with preserved ejection fraction. Heart Fail Clin. 2014;10(3):377–88. doi: 10.1016/j.hfc.2014.04.003. PMID: 24975902.

Gut Health, Intestinal Permeability, and Mineral Absorption

25. Coudray C, Demigné C, Rayssiguier Y. Effects of dietary fibers on magnesium absorption in animals and humans. Journal of Nutrition. 2003;133(1):1–4. doi:10.1093/jn/133.1.1. Factors affecting magnesium absorption in the GI tract.

26. Lönnerdal B. Dietary factors influencing zinc absorption. Journal of Nutrition. 2000;130(5S Suppl):1378S-1383S. doi:10.1093/jn/130.5.1378S. Dietary factors that enhance or inhibit zinc absorption.

27. Macura B, Kiecka A, Szczepanik M. Intestinal permeability disturbances: causes, diseases and therapy. Clinical and Experimental Medicine. 2024;24(1):232. doi:10.1007/s10238-024-01496-9. Comprehensive review of leaky gut causes, consequences, and treatments.

28. Camilleri M. Leaky gut: mechanisms, measurement and clinical implications in humans. Gut. 2019;68:1516–1526. doi:10.1136/gutjnl-2019-318427. Clinical review of intestinal permeability measurement and significance.

29. Ghorbani Z, Shoaibinobarian N, et al. Reinforcing gut integrity: probiotics, synbiotics, and prebiotics on intestinal permeability markers. Pharmacological Research. 2025;216:107780. doi:10.1016/j.phrs.2025.107780. Meta-analysis showing pro/prebiotics help alleviate leaky gut.

PART III: WHEN SYMPTOMS SPEAK

Pain, Cramps, and Muscle Function

30. Garrison SR, Korownyk CS, Kolber MR, et al. Magnesium for skeletal muscle cramps. Cochrane Database of Systematic Reviews. 2020;9:CD009402. doi:10.1002/14651858.CD009402.pub3. Meta-analysis of 11 RCTs (n=735): Mg unlikely to benefit older adults with cramps; may help pregnancy cramps. [Note: Evidence quality low-moderate.]

31. Sebo P, Cerutti B, Haller DM. Effect of magnesium therapy on nocturnal leg cramps: systematic review with meta-analysis. Family Practice. 2014;31(1):7–19. doi:10.1093/fampra/cmt065. 7 RCTs (n=361): Mg may have small effect in pregnant women but not general population.

32. Tarsitano MG, et al. Effects of magnesium supplementation on muscle soreness in different physical activities: a systematic review. Journal of Translational Medicine. 2024;22:629. doi:10.1186/s12967-024-05434-x. MgS reduced muscle soreness, improved recovery; athletes need 10–20% higher Mg than sedentary.

Sleep Disorders and Insomnia

33. Mah J, Pitre T. Oral magnesium supplementation for insomnia in older adults: systematic review & meta-analysis. BMC Complementary Medicine and Therapies. 2021;21:125. doi:10.1186/s12906-021-03297-z. 3 RCTs (n=151): Mg reduced sleep onset latency by 17.36 min (p=0.0006); total sleep time improved 16 min (NS).

34. Arab A, Rafie N, Amani R, Shirani F. The role of magnesium in sleep health: a systematic review. Biological Trace Element Research. 2023;201(1):121–128. doi:10.1007/s12011-022-03162-1. 9 studies (n=7,582): Association between Mg status and sleep quality in observational studies.

35. Held K, et al. Oral Mg2+ supplementation reverses age-related neuroendocrine and sleep EEG changes. Pharmacopsychiatry. 2002;35(4):135–143. doi:10.1055/s-2002-33195. Mg supplementation improved slow-wave sleep and normalized neuroendocrine markers.

36. Abbasi B, Kimiagar M, Sadeghniiat K, et al. Effect of magnesium supplementation on primary insomnia in elderly. Journal of Research in Medical Sciences. 2012;17(12):1161–1169. RCT showing Mg improved ISI scores, sleep efficiency, melatonin, and reduced cortisol.

Energy Production and Fatigue

37. Yamanaka R, Tabata S, Shindo Y, et al. Mitochondrial Mg2+ homeostasis decides cellular energy metabolism. Scientific Reports. 2016;6:30027. doi:10.1038/srep30027. Mitochondrial magnesium regulates ATP production.

38. Feeney KA, Hansen LL, Putker M, et al. Daily magnesium fluxes regulate cellular timekeeping and energy balance. Nature. 2016;532(7599):375–379. doi:10.1038/nature17407. Landmark study: Mg fluxes essential for cellular energy regulation.

Brain, Mood, and Mental Clarity

39. Moabedi M, Aliakbari M, Erfanian S, Milajerdi A. Magnesium supplementation beneficially affects depression: systematic review and meta-analysis. Frontiers in Psychiatry. 2023;14:1333261. doi:10.3389/fpsyt.2023.1333261. 7 RCTs (n=325): Significant depression reduction (SMD: -0.919).

40. Boyle NB, Lawton C, Dye L. Effects of magnesium supplementation on subjective anxiety and stress—systematic review. Nutrients. 2017;9(5):429. doi:10.3390/nu9050429. 18 studies: Beneficial effects in mildly anxious populations.

41. Wang J, Um P, Dickerman BA, Liu J. Zinc, magnesium, selenium and depression: evidence and mechanisms. Nutrients. 2018;10(5):584. doi:10.3390/nu10050584. Comprehensive review of mineral-depression relationships.

42. Slutsky I, Abumaria N, Wu LJ, et al. Enhancement of learning and memory by elevating brain magnesium. Neuron. 2010;65(2):165–177. doi:10.1016/j.neuron.2009.12.026. Landmark study: Brain Mg enhances learning/memory via synaptic plasticity.

43. Gutema BT, Sorrie MB, Megersa ND, et al. Effects of iron supplementation on cognitive development in school-age children: meta-analysis. PLOS One. 2023;18(6):e0287703. doi:10.1371/journal.pone.0287703. 13 RCTs: Iron improves intelligence (SMD 0.46), attention (0.44), memory (0.44).

Cardiovascular Health and Blood Pressure

44. Filippini T, Violi F, D'Amico R, Vinceti M. Effect of potassium supplementation on blood pressure in hypertensives: meta-analysis. International Journal of Cardiology. 2017;230:127–135. doi:10.1016/j.ijcard.2016.12.048. K decreases SBP by 4.48 mmHg and DBP by 2.96 mmHg.

45. Zhang X, Li Y, Del Gobbo LC, et al. Effects of magnesium supplementation on blood pressure: meta-analysis. Hypertension. 2016;68(2):324–333. doi:10.1161/HYPERTENSIONAHA.116.07664. Mg reduces SBP by 2.00 mmHg and DBP by 1.78 mmHg.

46. Appel LJ, Moore TJ, Obarzanek E, et al. Clinical trial of dietary patterns on blood pressure (DASH). New England Journal of Medicine. 1997;336(16):1117–1124. doi:10.1056/NEJM199704173361601. DASH reduced BP by ~11.4/approximately 5.5 mmHg in hypertensive participants.

Hormones and Thyroid Function

47. Huwiler VV, et al. Selenium supplementation in Hashimoto thyroiditis: meta-analysis. Thyroid. 2024;34(3):295–313. doi:10.1089/thy.2023.0556. 35 studies: Selenium reduces TSH and TPOAb.

48. Zuo Y, Li Y, Gu X, Lei Z. Selenium levels and autoimmune thyroid disease: meta-analysis. Annals of Palliative Medicine. 2021;10(4):4398–4408. doi:10.21037/apm-21-449. 17 RCTs: Se reduces FT3, FT4, and TPOAb.

49. Zimmermann MB, Boelaert K. Iodine deficiency and thyroid disorders. The Lancet Diabetes & Endocrinology. 2015;3(4):286–295. doi:10.1016/S2213-8587(14)70225-6. Landmark review on iodine's role in thyroid function.

Immune Function and Inflammation

50. Jafari A, et al. Zinc supplementation and immune factors: meta-analysis. Critical Reviews in Food Science and Nutrition. 2022;62(11):3023–3041. doi:10.1080/10408398.2020.1862048. 35 RCTs (n=1995): Zn reduces CRP, increases CD4.

51. Sanna A, Firinu D, Zavattari P, Valera P. Zinc status and autoimmunity: meta-analysis. Nutrients. 2018;10(1):68. doi:10.3390/nu10010068. 62 studies: Lower zinc in autoimmune patients.

52. Wessels I, Maywald M, Rink L. Zinc as a gatekeeper of immune function. Nutrients. 2017;9(12):1286. doi:10.3390/nu9121286. Zinc's essential role in immune cell development.

53. Hemilä H, et al. (2017). Zinc acetate lozenges may improve recovery from common colds. Open Forum Infectious Diseases. 4(2):ofx059. doi:10.1093/ofid/ofx059. Day-5 recovery 70% zinc vs 27% placebo.

Exercise and Athletic Performance

54. Zhang H, Wang R, Guo S, et al. Lower serum magnesium concentration and higher 24-h urinary magnesium excretion despite higher dietary magnesium intake in athletes: a systematic review and meta-analysis. Food Science and Human Wellness. 2023;12(5):1471–1480. doi:10.1016/j.fshw.2023.02.015. Athletes have lower serum Mg (-0.04 mmol/L) despite higher intake (+52 mg/day) due to increased urinary excretion.

55. Chen HY, Cheng FC, Pan HC, et al. Magnesium enhances exercise performance via increasing glucose availability. PLOS One. 2014;9(1):e85486. doi:10.1371/journal.pone.0085486. Mg improves glucose availability in brain, muscle, blood during exercise.

56. Volpe SL. Magnesium and the Athlete. Current Sports Medicine Reports. 2015;14(4):279–283. doi:10.1249/JSR.0000000000000178. Review: Athletes may need 10–20% more Mg than sedentary individuals.

57. Nielsen FH, Lukaski HC. Update on the relationship between magnesium and exercise. Magnesium Research. 2006;19(3):180–189. Physical activity increases Mg requirements; marginal deficiency impairs performance.

Hair, Skin, and Nails

58. Treister-Goltzman Y, Yarza S, Peleg R. Iron deficiency and nonscarring alopecia in women: systematic review and meta-analysis. Skin Appendage Disorders. 2022;8(2):83–92. doi:10.1159/000519952. 36 studies (n=10,029): Women with hair loss had ferritin 18.5 ng/mL lower; 21% prevalence of low ferritin.

59. Moeinvaziri M, Mansoori P, et al. Iron status in diffuse telogen hair loss among women. Acta Dermatovenerologica Croatica. 2009;17(4):279–284. Ferritin ≤30 ng/mL: OR 21.0 for telogen hair loss.

60. Wang R, Lin J, et al. Micronutrients and Androgenetic Alopecia: A Systematic Review. Molecular Nutrition & Food Research. 2024;68(22):e2400652. doi:10.1002/mnfr.202400652. 49 studies: Vitamin B, D, iron, zinc critical for hair growth.

61. Chang HC, Chang YS. Association between serum zinc levels and androgenetic alopecia: a systematic review and meta-analysis. Journal of Cosmetic Dermatology. 2022;21(4):1774–1777. doi:10.1111/jocd.14564. Lower zinc associated with male pattern hair loss.

62. Dhaher SA, Yacoub AA, Jacob AA. Estimation of zinc and iron levels in women with androgenetic alopecia. Indian Journal of Dermatology. 2018;63(5):369–374. doi:10.4103/ijd.IJD_624_16. Serum zinc significantly lower in women with hair loss (65.6 vs 128.4 µg/dL, $p<0.05$).

63. Wu R, Li Y, Peng H, et al. Serum trace elements and alopecia areata: systematic review and meta-analysis. Journal of Cosmetic Dermatology. 2025;24(1):e16740. doi:10.1111/jocd.16740. Zn and vitamin D deficiencies significantly associated with alopecia areata risk.

PART IV: MAKING IT WORK

Chromium and Blood Sugar Regulation

64. Suksomboon N, Poolsup N, Yuwanakorn A. Systematic review and meta-analysis of the efficacy and safety of chromium supplementation in diabetes. Journal of Clinical Pharmacy and Therapeutics. 2014;39(3):292–306. doi:10.1111/jcpt.12147. 25 RCTs: Chromium reduced HbA1c (-0.55%), fasting glucose (-1.15 mmol/L) in diabetics; picolinate form most effective.

65. Asbaghi O, et al. Effects of chromium supplementation on glycemic control in patients with type 2 diabetes: meta-analysis. Pharmacological Research. 2020;161:105098. doi:10.1016/j.phrs.2020.105098. 28 RCTs: Cr reduced FPG (-19 mg/dL), HbA1c (-0.71%), HOMA-IR (-1.53). [Note: High heterogeneity; effects mainly in diabetics, not healthy subjects.]

Copper-Zinc Balance and Safety

66. Duncan A, Yacoubian C, Watson N, Morrison I. The risk of copper deficiency in patients prescribed zinc supplements. Journal of Clinical Pathology. 2015;68(9):723–725. doi:10.1136/jclinpath-2014-202837. 62% of patients prescribed zinc received doses sufficient to cause copper deficiency; awareness of this risk was lacking.

67. Duncan A, Morrison I. Iatrogenic copper deficiency: Risks and cautions with zinc prescribing. British Journal of Clinical Pharmacology. 2023;89(9):2825–2829. doi:10.1111/bcp.15749. 50% of zinc-induced copper deficiency cases were previously undiagnosed; recommends guidelines revision for zinc prescribing.

68. Hoffman HN, Phyliky RL, Fleming CR. Zinc-induced copper deficiency. Gastroenterology. 1988;94(2):508–512. doi:10.1016/0016-5085(88)90445-3. Landmark case: Anemia, leukopenia, neutropenia from high-dose zinc; copper absorption blocked until zinc eliminated.

Bone Health and Long-Term Maintenance

69. Weaver CM, Alexander DD, Boushey CJ, et al. Calcium plus vitamin D supplementation and fracture risk: NOF meta-analysis. Osteoporosis International. 2016;27(1):367–376. doi:10.1007/s00198-015-3386-5. 8 RCTs: 15% reduced total fractures (RR 0.85), 30% reduced hip fractures (RR 0.70).

70. Dawson-Hughes B, Harris SS, Krall EA, Dallal GE. Effect of calcium and vitamin D supplementation on bone density. New England Journal of Medicine. 1997;337(10):670–676. doi:10.1056/NEJM199709043371003. Landmark RCT: Ca+D reduce bone loss and fractures in older adults.

Vitamin D Status and Guidelines

71. Forrest KY, Stuhldreher WL. Prevalence of vitamin D deficiency in US adults. Nutrition Research. 2011;31(1):48–54. doi:10.1016/j.nutres.2010.12.001. NHANES 2005–2006: 41.6% deficiency (≤20 ng/mL).

72. Holick MF, et al. Evaluation, treatment, and prevention of vitamin D deficiency: an Endocrine Society clinical practice guideline. JCEM. 2011;96(7):1911–1930. doi:10.1210/jc.2011-0385. Treatment protocol: 50,000 IU weekly ×8 weeks, then 1,500–2,000 IU/day. Updated and replaced by: Demay MB, Pittas AG, Bikle DD, et al. Vitamin D for the prevention of disease: an Endocrine Society clinical practice guideline. JCEM. 2024;109(8):1907–1947. doi:10.1210/clinem/dgae290, which advises against routine screening and above-RDA supplementation in generally healthy adults under 75.

Prevalence of Mineral Deficiencies

73. Rosanoff A, Weaver CM, Rude RK. Suboptimal magnesium status in the United States. Nutrition Reviews. 2012;70(3):153–164. doi:10.1111/j.1753-4887.2011.00465.x. Widespread subclinical Mg deficiency in US population.

74. Wessells KR, Brown KH. Estimating global prevalence of zinc deficiency. PLOS One. 2012;7(11):e50568. doi:10.1371/journal.pone.0050568. 17.3% of world population at risk for zinc deficiency.

75. Prasad AS. Discovery of human zinc deficiency: impact on human health and disease. Advances in Nutrition. 2013;4(2):176–190. doi:10.3945/an.112.003210. Historical perspective on zinc deficiency discovery.

Glucose Metabolism and Diabetes Prevention

76. Daneshvar M, et al. Effect of zinc supplementation on glycemic biomarkers: umbrella meta-analysis. Diabetology & Metabolic Syndrome. 2024;16:124. doi:10.1186/s13098-024-01366-0. Zn reduces FBS (-13.58 mg/dL), HOMA-IR (-0.52), HbA1c (-0.35%).

77. Barbagallo M, Dominguez LJ. Magnesium and type 2 diabetes. World Journal of Diabetes. 2015;6(10):1152–1157. doi:10.4239/wjd.v6.i10.1152. Mg role in insulin secretion, action, and glucose metabolism.

78. Felitti VJ, Anda RF, Nordenberg D, Williamson DF, Spitz AM, Edwards V, Koss MP, Marks JS. Relationship of childhood abuse and household dysfunction to many of the leading causes of death in adults. The Adverse Childhood Experiences (ACE) Study. Am J Prev Med. 1998;14(4):245–258. doi:10.1016/S0749-3797(98)00017-8. PMID: 9635069.

79. Alzahrani H. Assessment of Vitamin B12 Efficacy on Cognitive Memory Function and Depressive Symptoms: A Systematic Review and Meta-Analysis. Cureus. 2024;16(11):e73350. doi: 10.7759/cureus.73350.

80. Soriano-Gonzalez R, Ramirez-Olea H, Gonzalez-Soltero R, Chavez-Santoscoy RA. The biological relationship among depression, vitamins B9, B12, and D, and genetic variants: a systematic review. Front Nutr. 2025;12:1690378. doi: 10.3389/fnut.2025.1690378.

81. Ghaemi S, Zeraattalab-Motlagh S, Jayedi A, Shab-Bidar S. The effect of vitamin D supplementation on depression: a systematic review and dose—response meta-analysis of randomized controlled trials. Psychol Med. 2024;54(14):3463–3474. doi: 10.1017/S0033291724001697.

82. Wang L, Su S, Liu Y. Meta-analysis of the effect of vitamin D on depression. Front Psychiatry. 2025;16:1622796. doi: 10.3389/fpsyt.2025.1622796.

83. Thys-Jacobs S, Starkey P, Bernstein D, Tian J. Calcium carbonate and the premenstrual syndrome: effects on premenstrual and menstrual symptoms. Premenstrual Syndrome Study Group. Am J Obstet Gynecol. 1998;179(2):444-452. doi: 10.1016/s0002-9378(98)70377-1. PMID: 9731851.

84. Walker AF, De Souza MC, Vickers MF, Abeyasekera S, Collins ML, Trinca LA. Magnesium supplementation alleviates premenstrual symptoms of fluid retention. J Womens Health. 1998;7(9):1157-1165. doi: 10.1089/jwh.1998.7.1157. PMID: 9861593.

85. Beck MA, Shi Q, Morris VC, Levander OA. Rapid genomic evolution of a non-virulent coxsackievirus B3 in selenium-deficient mice results in selection of identical virulent isolates. Nat Med. 1995;1(5):433-436. doi: 10.1038/nm0595-433. PMID: 7585090.

86. Martineau AR, Jolliffe DA, Hooper RL, et al. Vitamin D supplementation to prevent acute respiratory tract infections: systematic review and meta-analysis of individual participant data. BMJ. 2017;356:i6583. doi: 10.1136/bmj.i6583. PMID: 28202713.

87. Davis DR, Epp MD, Riordan HD. Changes in USDA food composition data for 43 garden crops, 1950 to 1999. J Am Coll Nutr. 2004;23(6):669-682. doi: 10.1080/07315724.2004.10719409. PMID: 15637215.

88. Mahmood A, FitzGerald AJ, Marchbank T, et al. Zinc carnosine, a health food supplement that stabilises small bowel integrity and stimulates gut repair processes. Gut. 2007;56(2):168-175. doi: 10.1136/gut.2006.099929. PMID: 16777920.

89. Verdon F, Burnand B, Stubi CL, et al. Iron supplementation for unexplained fatigue in non-anaemic women: double blind randomised placebo controlled trial. BMJ. 2003;326(7399):1124. doi: 10.1136/bmj.326.7399.1124. PMID: 12763985.

90. Krayenbuehl PA, Battegay E, Breymann C, Furrer J, Schulthess G. Intravenous iron for the treatment of fatigue in nonanemic, premenopausal women with low serum ferritin concentration. Blood. 2011;118(12):3222-3227. doi: 10.1182/blood-2011-04-346304. PMID: 21705493.

91. Dibaba DT, Xun P, Song Y, Rosanoff A, Shechter M, He K. The effect of magnesium supplementation on blood pressure in individuals with insulin resistance, prediabetes, or noncommunicable chronic diseases: a meta-analysis of randomized controlled trials. Am J Clin Nutr. 2017;106(3):921-929. doi: 10.3945/ajcn.117.155291. PMID: 28724644.

92. Telford RD, Sly GJ, Hahn AG, Cunningham RB, Bryant C, Smith JA. Footstrike is the major cause of hemolysis during running. J Appl Physiol (1985). 2003;94(1):38-42. doi: 10.1152/japplphysiol.00631.2001. PMID: 12391035.

93. Trost LB, Bergfeld WF, Calogeras E. The diagnosis and treatment of iron deficiency and its potential relationship to hair loss. J Am Acad Dermatol. 2006;54(5):824-844. doi: 10.1016/j.jaad.2005.11.1104. PMID: 16635664.

94. Hochman LG, Scher RK, Meyerson MS. Brittle nails: response to daily biotin supplementation. Cutis. 1993;51(4):303-305. PMID: 8477615.

95. Lindenbaum J, Healton EB, Savage DG, et al. Neuropsychiatric disorders caused by cobalamin deficiency in the absence of anemia or macrocytosis. N Engl J Med. 1988;318(26):1720-1728. doi: 10.1056/NEJM198806303182604. PMID: 3374544.

Note: Guidelines and recommendations may be updated; clinicians should consult current practice guidelines. For additional reading, search PubMed using relevant keywords.

APPENDIX B—MINERAL PROFILES

How to Use These Profiles

This is reference material. Think of it like a mini-encyclopedia you look things up in when you need them. You don't have to read the whole thing.

Most people only care about 1–3 minerals. Which ones matter for you depends on how you feel, what you eat, what medications you take, and what your test results show.

Got muscle cramps and can't sleep? **Read Magnesium.**

Exhausted all the time? **Read Iron.**

Always getting sick? **Read Zinc.**

Doctor said you're low on something? **Read that one.**

Just curious? **Skim the Bottom Line section of each mineral.**

You can skip the minerals that don't apply to you. One less thing to stress about.

Jump to a Mineral

Big 5	Important	Rare Deficiency	Non-Essential
Magnesium	**Selenium**	**Manganese**	**Fluoride**
Iron	**Potassium**	**Molybdenum**	**Boron**
Zinc	**Chromium**	**Phosphorus**	**Silicon**
Calcium	**Copper**	**Sodium**	**Lithium (trace)**
Iodine		**Sulfur**	

THE BIG 5

Most Common Deficiencies—If you only read five profiles, read these.

Mg Magnesium

Magnesium is involved in over 300 chemical processes in your body. It helps muscles relax, calms your nervous system, makes energy, controls blood sugar, and builds bones. About half of Americans don't get enough. Blood tests don't catch deficiency until it's severe, so you can feel terrible while your tests look normal.

What It Does in Your Body

Makes energy. Every cell runs on ATP. Your body cannot make this fuel without magnesium.

Relaxes muscles. Calcium makes muscles contract; magnesium makes them relax. Without enough, muscles stay partly contracted causing cramps and tension.

Calms nerves. Acts like a brake for your nervous system, blocking signals that keep nerves fired up.

Controls blood sugar. Your body needs magnesium to make insulin work properly.

Builds bones. About 60% of your body's magnesium is stored in bones.

How Much You Need

Group	Amount
Men	**400–420 mg daily**
Women	**310–320 mg daily**
Pregnant	**350–360 mg daily**
Max from supplements	**350 mg daily**

Top Food Sources

Food	Serving	Amount
Pumpkin seeds	**1 oz**	**156 mg**
Chia seeds	**1 oz**	**95 mg**
Almonds	**1 oz**	**80 mg**
Spinach, cooked	**½ cup**	**78 mg**
Dark chocolate (70–85%)	**1 oz**	**64 mg**
Black beans	**½ cup**	**60 mg**

Signs of Deficiency

Common signs:

- Muscle cramps, twitches, or spasms (especially legs at night)
- Restless legs when trying to sleep
- Anxiety or feeling on edge

- Trouble falling asleep or staying asleep
- Frequent headaches or migraines
- Constipation that won't go away
- Severe PMS or period cramps
- Chocolate cravings

Severe deficiency:

Irregular heartbeat, numbness or tingling, seizures

Should You Supplement?

Yes, if you have: Any symptoms above, digestive disorders, diabetes, chronic stress, heavy sweating, or are over 65.

Who else is at risk: People taking PPIs (Prilosec, Nexium), diuretics, or eating mostly processed foods.

How to take it: Start with 200–300 mg at bedtime. Magnesium helps with sleep, so evening is best. Give it 2–4 weeks.

> **Critical Safety Information**
>
> Magnesium is very safe for most people. The main side effect is diarrhea from taking too much—lower your dose if this happens. Exception: Kidney disease. If you have kidney disease, talk to your doctor first. Damaged kidneys cannot remove extra magnesium.

Drug Interactions:

- Antibiotics (doxycycline, Cipro): Take 2 hours apart
- Bisphosphonates: Take 2 hours apart
- Blood pressure meds: May work better—tell your doctor

Best Supplemental Forms

Magnesium glycinate—BEST CHOICE

Well absorbed, does not cause diarrhea, best for anxiety, sleep, and muscle problems.

Magnesium citrate—Well absorbed, more likely to cause loose stools. Good if you need help with constipation.

Magnesium malate—Good for energy and chronic fatigue.

Magnesium threonate—Best for brain function and memory. More expensive.

> **AVOID**
>
> Magnesium oxide—Poorly absorbed (only 4%). Common in cheap supplements. Mostly causes diarrhea.

Fe Iron

Iron carries oxygen in your blood. Without enough iron, your cells are starving for oxygen—explaining why iron deficiency makes you exhausted, out of breath, mentally foggy, cold, and unable to think straight. Iron deficiency is the most common nutritional deficiency worldwide. But too much iron is toxic. Your body has no way to get rid of extra iron. This is the mineral where you really need to test, not guess.

What It Does in Your Body

Carries oxygen. Iron is the central part of hemoglobin. Without it, your blood can't do its most basic job.

Makes energy. Iron-containing enzymes turn food into usable energy.

Runs your immune system. White blood cells need iron to multiply when fighting infection.

Makes brain chemicals. Iron helps produce dopamine, serotonin, and norepinephrine.

How Much You Need

Group	Amount
Men (19+)	**8 mg daily**
Women (19–50)	**18 mg daily**
Women (51+)	**8 mg daily**
Pregnant	**27 mg daily**
Vegetarians	**Multiply by 1.8**
Max safe	**45 mg daily**

Top Food Sources

Animal Sources (better absorbed)	Serving	Amount
Oysters	**3 oz**	**8 mg**
Beef liver	**3 oz**	**5 mg**
Beef	**3 oz**	**2–3 mg**

Plant Sources (less absorbed)	Serving	Amount
Fortified cereal	**1 serving**	**18 mg**
White beans	**1 cup**	**8 mg**
Lentils	**½ cup**	**3.3 mg**

Absorption tip: Eat plant-based iron with vitamin C to increase absorption. Avoid tea, coffee, and calcium with iron-rich meals.

Signs of Deficiency

Early deficiency (low iron stores, not anemic yet):

- Fatigue and low energy despite sleeping enough
- Hard to concentrate, brain fog
- Cold hands and feet
- Restless leg syndrome
- Craving ice, dirt, or other non-food items

Iron-deficiency anemia (more advanced):

- Extreme exhaustion affecting daily life
- Pale skin, nail beds, and inner eyelids
- Shortness of breath with light activity
- Brittle nails or spoon-shaped nails
- Hair loss

Should You Supplement?

GET TESTED FIRST

This is required with iron. Request a complete blood count (CBC) and ferritin level. Don't take iron "just in case"—iron is one mineral where more is definitely not better.

Take supplements if: Ferritin below 30 ng/mL (even if hemoglobin normal), documented anemia, or pregnant.

Higher risk if: Heavy periods, pregnant/breastfeeding, vegetarian/vegan, digestive disorders, frequent blood donation, endurance athlete, long-term PPI use.

Don't take if: You're a man or postmenopausal woman with normal levels, or have hemochromatosis.

Critical Safety Information

Iron is one of the leading causes of poisoning deaths in children. Just 1–2 grams can be fatal to a small child. Keep supplements locked away. Hemochromatosis: Some people have a genetic condition causing too much iron absorption. If you have a family history, get tested before taking iron. Don't take during active infections—bacteria need iron to multiply.

Drug Interactions:

- Thyroid medications (levothyroxine): Separate by 4+ hours
- Antibiotics: Separate by 2–4 hours
- Calcium supplements: Take separately

Best Supplemental Forms

Iron bisglycinate (chelated iron)—BEST TOLERATED

Highly absorbable, very gentle on stomach, much less constipation and nausea. Often called "gentle iron."

Ferrous sulfate—Most commonly prescribed, inexpensive. Most likely to cause constipation and nausea.

Ferrous gluconate—Better tolerated with less constipation.

AVOID

Time-release or enteric-coated iron—These don't dissolve until past where iron is absorbed. Poorly absorbed despite marketing.

Tips

Take on empty stomach with vitamin C for best absorption. If nausea, take with food. Try every-other-day dosing—research shows better absorption and fewer side effects. Expect dark stools (this is normal).

Zn Zinc

Zinc is essential for immune function, wound healing, taste and smell, skin health, and cell division. When you don't have enough, your immune system fails (frequent infections), wounds heal slowly, food tastes bland, your skin breaks out, and you lose hair. But too much zinc blocks copper absorption, creating a new deficiency. The sweet spot: 8–11 mg daily from food, supplement with 15–25 mg if needed, and if you take more than 30 mg, add 1–2 mg of copper.

What It Does in Your Body

Runs your immune system. Required for immune cells to develop and function.

Heals wounds. Necessary for cells to divide, make collagen, and repair tissue.

Maintains taste and smell. Deficiency makes food taste like cardboard.

Supports male fertility. Essential for testosterone and healthy sperm.

Keeps skin healthy. Controls oil production and reduces inflammation.

How Much You Need

Group	Amount
Men (19+)	**11 mg daily**
Women (19+)	**8 mg daily**
Pregnant	**11 mg daily**
Max safe	**40 mg daily**

Top Food Sources

Food	Serving	Amount
Oysters	**3 oz**	**74 mg (!)**
Beef	**3 oz**	**7 mg**
Alaska king crab	**3 oz**	**6.5 mg**
Pumpkin seeds	**1 oz**	**2.2 mg**

Note: Plant zinc is only absorbed at 10–20% vs 25–50% from animal sources. Soaking, sprouting, or fermenting grains/beans improves absorption.

Signs of Deficiency

• Frequent infections—colds, flu, respiratory infections

• Wounds heal slowly

• Loss of taste or smell, food tastes bland

• Acne or other skin problems

• Hair loss or thinning

• White spots on fingernails

If you're always catching whatever's going around and cuts take forever to heal, think zinc.

Should You Supplement?

Consider if: Frequent infections, vegetarian/vegan, pregnant/breastfeeding, elderly, digestive disorders, heavy alcohol use.

How much: 15–25 mg daily for general immune support.

For acute cold: Zinc lozenges (13–23 mg) started within 24 hours may reduce cold length. Use 5–7 days max.

> **CRITICAL: Balance with copper**
>
> **If taking more than 25–30 mg zinc daily for any length of time, add 1–2 mg copper. The ideal ratio is roughly 15:1 zinc to copper.**

> **Safety Information**
>
> High-dose zinc (50+ mg daily long-term) can cause: Copper deficiency (leading to anemia), immune suppression (the opposite of what you want!), reduced HDL cholesterol. Zinc nasal sprays and gels: Do NOT use them. They've been linked to permanent loss of smell. Stick to pills or lozenges only.

Best Supplemental Forms

Zinc picolinate—BEST CHOICE

Highly absorbable, well-tolerated.

Zinc citrate, zinc gluconate, zinc glycinate—All well absorbed, good options.

> **AVOID**
>
> Zinc oxide—Poorly absorbed. Common in cheap multivitamins.

Ca Calcium

> Calcium isn't just about bones. While 99% lives in your skeleton, that remaining 1% controls your heartbeat, helps muscles contract, allows nerves to send messages, and helps blood clot. Here's what most people miss: Most Americans get too much calcium from supplements while not getting enough from food. High-dose supplements have been linked to kidney stones, constipation, and possibly heart problems. Bone health requires more than calcium—you also need magnesium, vitamin D, vitamin K2, and weight-bearing exercise.

How Much You Need

Group	Amount
Adults (19–50)	**1,000 mg daily**
Women 51+ / Men 71+	**1,200 mg daily**
Max safe	**2,000–2,500 mg daily**

Top Food Sources

Food	Serving	Amount
Plain low-fat yogurt	**1 cup**	**415 mg**
Sardines with bones	**3 oz**	**325 mg**
Cheddar cheese	**1.5 oz**	**307 mg**
Milk	**1 cup**	**300 mg**
Collard greens, cooked	**1 cup**	**268 mg**

Your body can only absorb about 500 mg at once—spread intake throughout the day.

Signs of Deficiency

Early (often missed): Muscle cramps/spasms, numbness/tingling in fingers and toes, brittle nails, tooth decay

Advanced: Bone pain, fractures from minor falls, osteoporosis, abnormal heart rhythms

Should You Supplement?

Food sources are always better because they come with other bone-supporting nutrients.

If you do supplement: Split dose (body absorbs 500 mg max at once), take with meals, ensure adequate vitamin D, choose calcium citrate if over 50 or on acid blockers. **Do not exceed 2,000–2,500 mg total daily intake; high doses are linked to kidney stones.**

A note on calcium supplements and heart health

Whether calcium supplements increase cardiovascular risk is a contested question in the medical literature. Several meta-analyses (Bolland 2010, Myung 2021) have found roughly 15–25% increased cardiovascular event risk in healthy postmenopausal women taking 1,000 mg/day or more — a signal that persists with concurrent vitamin D. Other meta-analyses have found no significant effect, and the National Osteoporosis Foundation and American Society for Preventive Cardiology issued a joint guideline finding no association in generally healthy adults.

The proposed mechanism: supplement doses cause sharp post-dose serum calcium spikes that don't happen with food calcium. Mendelian randomization studies — which test causality through genetic variation — also link circulating calcium to cardiovascular risk.

Practical takeaway: get calcium from food first, keep any supplemental doses under 500 mg at a time, and discuss with your doctor if you have cardiovascular risk factors. The signal in the literature is strongest at 1,000 mg/day or more.

Balance with magnesium. Aim for 2:1 ratio (calcium to magnesium). Too much calcium without adequate magnesium causes cramps and constipation.

Best Supplemental Forms

Calcium citrate—Better absorbed, especially for older adults or those with low stomach acid. Can take with or without food.

Calcium carbonate—Cheaper, more calcium per pill. Must take with food. Works fine if you have normal stomach acid.

> **AVOID**
>
> Calcium from oyster shell, bone meal, or dolomite—Unless verified free of lead contamination.

I Iodine

> Iodine is essential for thyroid hormone production. Thyroid hormones control your metabolism—the rate at which every cell operates. Without enough iodine, you feel tired, cold, foggy, and constipated. Hair falls out. You gain weight easily. Deficiency is making a comeback because people use sea salt and Himalayan pink salt (no iodine) instead of iodized salt, and are cutting back on dairy and bread.

How Much You Need

Group	Amount
Adults	**150 mcg daily**
Pregnant	**220 mcg daily**
Breastfeeding	**290 mcg daily**
Max safe	**1,100 mcg daily**

Top Food Sources

Food	Serving	Amount
Seaweed (varies wildly)	**1 sheet**	**16–2,900 mcg**
Cod	**3 oz**	**99 mcg**
Iodized salt	**¼ tsp**	**71 mcg**
Milk	**1 cup**	**56–96 mcg**

Important: Sea salt, kosher salt, and Himalayan pink salt contain almost no iodine. Only iodized table salt is reliable.

Signs of Deficiency

Early/mild: Fatigue, weight gain, feeling cold, dry skin/hair, constipation, brain fog, heavy/irregular periods

Moderate: Goiter (swelling at base of neck), hair loss, depression

In pregnancy: Increased risk of miscarriage, developmental disabilities in baby

Should You Supplement?

If pregnant/breastfeeding: Take prenatal with 150–220 mcg iodine (check label—not all include it).

For everyone else: If you use iodized salt and eat seafood/dairy/eggs, you're probably fine. If you avoid all these, supplementation makes sense.

Standard dose: 150 mcg daily is safe and appropriate.

> **Be cautious with high-dose iodine (500+ mcg)**
>
> Despite marketing claims about "iodine loading," high intake can trigger or worsen thyroid problems.

If you have Hashimoto's or Graves' disease: Work with your endocrinologist before supplementing.

Seaweed is unpredictable. Some kelp contains milligrams per serving—easily exceeding safe limits.

Best Supplemental Forms

Potassium iodide—Most common, well-absorbed. Look for ~150 mcg per dose.

Kelp supplements—Wildly variable iodine content. Hard to dose accurately. Not recommended.

Important But Less Common

These matter, but deficiency happens less often or advice is straightforward.

Se Selenium

> Selenium acts as a powerful protector against cell damage, supports immunity, and regulates thyroid hormones. The catch: The safe zone between too little and too much is narrow. Too little means weakened immunity and thyroid problems. Too much (usually from over-supplementation) causes hair loss, brittle nails, and nerve damage. Most Americans get adequate selenium from food.

How Much You Need: Adults: 55 mcg daily | Max safe: 400 mcg daily

Top Food Sources: Brazil nuts (1 nut): 68–91 mcg (varies dramatically) | Yellowfin tuna (3 oz): 92 mcg | Halibut (3 oz): 47 mcg

Should You Supplement?

Most Americans don't need supplements. Consider 50–200 mcg daily if you have Hashimoto's thyroiditis (research suggests it may help reduce antibodies), live in low-selenium area with vegan diet, or have documented deficiency.

> **More is NOT better**
>
> High doses (400+ mcg) have been linked to Type 2 diabetes risk. Symptoms of toxicity: garlic breath, hair loss, brittle nails, nerve damage. Brazil nuts are unpredictable. Eating 2–3 daily can provide excessive selenium. If you eat Brazil nuts regularly, skip supplements.

Best Form: Selenomethionine—The form found naturally in foods, well absorbed.

K Potassium

> Potassium is the mineral of blood pressure control and heart rhythm. It helps counteract sodium's blood pressure-raising effects and keeps your heart beating regularly. Most Americans get far too much sodium and far too little potassium. Unlike most minerals, potassium is best increased through food rather than supplements, because getting high-dose potassium wrong can stop your heart.

How Much You Need: Women: 2,600 mg daily | Men: 3,400 mg daily | Supplemental: Should not exceed 99 mg per dose without prescription

Top Food Sources: Baked potato with skin: 941 mg | Avocado: 708 mg | White beans (½ cup): 595 mg | Salmon (3 oz): 534 mg | Banana: 422 mg

Almost all whole foods contain potassium. Processed foods are stripped of potassium and loaded with sodium.

Who should NOT supplement potassium:

- People with chronic kidney disease
- Those taking potassium-sparing diuretics (spironolactone, amiloride)
- Anyone on ACE inhibitors or ARBs
- People with Addison's disease

Cr Chromium

> Chromium helps insulin do its job—moving sugar from bloodstream into cells. Without enough, insulin becomes less effective, leading to blood sugar roller coasters, energy crashes, and cravings. Most Americans don't get enough from diet, and stores decline with age.

How Much You Need: Men: 30–35 mcg daily | Women: 20–25 mcg daily

Signs of Deficiency

Blood sugar swings, intense sugar/carb cravings, energy crashes after meals, difficulty losing weight, brain fog

Best Forms

Chromium picolinate—Most researched, good absorption.

Chromium polynicotinate—Also well absorbed.

> **AVOID**
>
> Chromium chloride—Poor absorption.

Cu Copper

> Copper is the unsung hero of energy production and tissue repair. It helps make red blood cells, maintain healthy nerves and immune function, and form collagen. But copper must be in perfect balance with zinc and iron. Too little: anemia, weak blood vessels, immune problems. Too much: liver and nervous system damage. Most people don't need to supplement copper—they need to stop taking zinc without balancing it with copper.

How Much You Need: Adults: 900 mcg daily | Max safe: 10,000 mcg (10 mg) daily

Top Food Sources: Beef liver (3 oz): 12,400 mcg | Oysters (3 oz): 4,850 mcg | Cashews (1 oz): 622 mcg | Dark chocolate (1 oz): 501 mcg

Should You Supplement?

Most people should NOT supplement copper unless you have a diagnosed deficiency or are taking high-dose zinc.

> **Exception**
>
> **If you take more than 25–30 mg of zinc daily, balance with 1–2 mg copper. Ideal ratio: 15:1 zinc to copper.**

You Probably Don't Need to Worry

Deficiency is rare. These take care of themselves if you eat normal food.

Mn Manganese

> Essential for bone formation, wound healing, and metabolism. Your body contains only 10–20 mg total, but that tiny amount is critical.

The good news: Deficiency is extremely rare—it's in whole grains, nuts, legumes, and leafy greens.

The bad news: Too much manganese (from contaminated water or occupational exposure) is toxic to the brain.

Should you supplement? No. Unless you have a specific medical condition, there's no reason.

Mo Molybdenum

(It's muh-LIB-duh-num) Essential for life—activates enzymes that help detoxify sulfites. But dietary deficiency has been documented exactly once in medical history (a patient on long-term IV feeding). If you're eating food—any food—you're getting enough.

Should you supplement? No. Cross this one off your worry list.

P Phosphorus

In your bones, DNA, cell membranes, and energy molecules. Required for bone building and energy production.

The catch: You're almost certainly getting too much, not too little. Phosphorus is added to processed foods, sodas, and fast food in massive amounts. High intake—especially without adequate calcium—can weaken bones.

Should you supplement? Absolutely not. Focus on reducing excess from processed foods.

Na Sodium

Essential for fluid balance, nerve signaling, and muscle contraction. The problem isn't that sodium is bad—it's that most Americans consume 3,400 mg daily when we only need 500 mg and should stay under 2,300 mg.

Should you supplement? For most people: absolutely not. We get far too much already.

Exception: Athletes training for hours in hot conditions need to replace sodium lost through sweat.

S Sulfur

The forgotten mineral. Third most abundant in your body, essential for proteins, detoxification, and making glutathione (your master protective compound). No RDA because if you're eating enough protein, you're getting enough sulfur.

Should you supplement? No. Some people try MSM (1,000–3,000 mg) for joint pain—research is mixed but it's generally safe.

Other Minerals You've Heard About

Non-essential minerals with interesting evidence or lots of marketing.

F Fluoride

Strengthens tooth enamel, prevents cavities.

The controversy: One of the most contentious topics in public health. Critics worry about mass medication; proponents cite cavity prevention benefits.

Supplement? No. If you drink fluoridated water and use fluoride toothpaste, you're getting enough.

B Boron

Plays a role in bone health, wound healing, and metabolism of calcium, magnesium, and vitamin D.

Supplement? Probably not. Consider 3 mg daily if you have osteoporosis and are already addressing vitamin D, calcium, and magnesium. For arthritis, 3–6 mg daily is worth trying—low risk, potential benefit.

Si Silicon (Silica)

Present in connective tissues, bones, and skin. May play a role in collagen formation.

Supplement? Probably not unless targeting skin, hair, or nail health. Evidence for these uses is weak despite heavy marketing. For bone health, focus first on calcium, magnesium, vitamin D, and K2.

Li Lithium (Trace Amounts)

At prescription doses, treats bipolar disorder. At trace amounts, emerging research suggests benefits for brain health and mood.

The evidence: Regions with higher naturally occurring lithium in water have lower rates of suicide and psychiatric hospitalizations. Interesting but not definitive.

Supplement? Controversial. Some integrative practitioners recommend 300–1,000 mcg daily for mood support. Do NOT use instead of psychiatric treatment for bipolar disorder or severe depression.

When to Skip the Trend

Ask these questions before trying a "new" mineral:

- Is there an established deficiency disease in humans?
- Are there peer-reviewed human intervention trials?
- Is the supplement industry the primary source of information?
- What's the safety profile?
- Have the basics been covered first?

Red flags for hype:

- Claims about "boosting cellular energy" without specific mechanisms
- Testimonials but no clinical trials
- "Newly discovered" or "ancient secret" marketing
- No established recommended dose or upper limit
- Claims to treat or cure serious diseases

> **Bottom line**
>
> Most people should focus on the essential 14 minerals. Of the non-essential minerals, boron and low-dose lithium have the most interesting evidence. Everything else can be safely ignored unless you have a specific medical condition and are working with a knowledgeable practitioner.

14 essential minerals • Organized by what actually matters for you

Find mineral-rich foods quickly—by mineral, by food, or by budget

Remember

Whole foods are always better than supplements. The minerals in food come packaged with other nutrients that help your body absorb and use them properly.

The Magnificent Seven

If you only remember seven foods from this entire book, remember these:

Food	Serving	Key Minerals
Pumpkin Seeds	**1 oz (¼ cup)**	**Mg 156mg, Zn 2.2mg, Fe 2.5mg, Cu 0.4mg**
Oysters	**3 oz (6 medium)**	**Zn 74mg, Cu 4.8mg, Fe 8mg, Se 45mcg**
Spinach (cooked)	**1 cup**	**Mg 157mg, K 839mg, Fe 6.4mg, Ca 245mg**
Sardines (with bones)	**3 oz**	**Ca 325mg, Se 45mcg, P 417mg, K 365mg**
Dark Chocolate (70%+)	**1 oz**	**Mg 64mg, Fe 3.4mg, Cu 0.5mg, Mn 0.5mg**
Lentils (cooked)	**1 cup**	**Fe 6.6mg, K 731mg, Mg 71mg, Zn 2.5mg**
Brazil Nuts	**2 nuts**	**Se 192mcg, Mg 54mg, Cu 0.5mg, P 104mg**

Key: Mg = Magnesium, Zn = Zinc, Fe = Iron, Cu = Copper, Se = Selenium, Ca = Calcium, K = Potassium, P = Phosphorus, Mn = Manganese

Multi-Mineral All-Stars by Category

Looking up what you already eat? Find your food here.

Seeds & Nuts

Food	Serving	Key Minerals
Pumpkin seeds	1 oz	Mg 156mg, Zn 2.2mg, Fe 2.5mg
Hemp seeds	3 Tbsp	Mg 210mg, Zn 3mg, Fe 2.4mg
Chia seeds	1 oz	Mg 95mg, Ca 179mg, P 244mg
Almonds	1 oz	Mg 80mg, Ca 76mg, Mn 0.6mg
Cashews	1 oz	Mg 74mg, Zn 1.6mg, Cu 0.6mg
Sunflower seeds	1 oz	Mg 37mg, Se 22mcg, Cu 0.5mg
Brazil nuts	2 nuts	Se 192mcg, Mg 54mg, Cu 0.5mg

Leafy Greens

Food	Serving	Key Minerals
Spinach, cooked	1 cup	Mg 157mg, K 839mg, Fe 6.4mg
Swiss chard, cooked	1 cup	Mg 150mg, K 960mg, Fe 4mg
Beet greens, cooked	1 cup	Mg 98mg, K 1309mg, Fe 2.7mg
Collard greens, cooked	1 cup	Ca 268mg, K 222mg, Mn 0.8mg
Kale, cooked	1 cup	Ca 94mg, K 296mg, Mn 0.5mg

Beans & Legumes

Food	Serving	Key Minerals
White beans, cooked	1 cup	Fe 6.6mg, K 1004mg, Mg 113mg
Lentils, cooked	1 cup	Fe 6.6mg, K 731mg, Mg 71mg
Lima beans, cooked	1 cup	K 955mg, Mg 81mg, Fe 4.5mg
Chickpeas, cooked	1 cup	Fe 4.7mg, Zn 2.5mg, Cu 0.6mg
Black beans, cooked	1 cup	Fe 3.6mg, Mg 120mg, K 611mg

Seafood

Food	Key Minerals
Oysters (3 oz)	**Zn 74mg, Cu 4.8mg, Se 45mcg**
Sardines (3 oz)	**Ca 325mg, Se 45mcg, P 417mg**
Salmon (3 oz)	**Se 40mcg, K 534mg, P 218mg**
Crab (3 oz)	**Zn 6.5mg, Cu 1mg, Se 37mcg**
Shrimp (3 oz)	**Se 40mcg, Zn 1.4mg, Cu 0.2mg**

Dairy & Eggs

Food	Key Minerals
Yogurt, plain (1 cup)	**Ca 415mg, K 380mg, P 306mg**
Milk (1 cup)	**Ca 300mg, K 366mg, I 56–96mcg**
Cheddar (1.5 oz)	**Ca 307mg, Zn 1.5mg, P 216mg**
Cottage cheese (1 cup)	**Ca 138mg, Se 20mcg, P 358mg**
Egg (1 large)	**Se 15mcg, I 24mcg, P 99mg**

Vegetables

Food	Key Minerals
Baked potato w/skin	**K 941mg, Mg 48mg, Fe 1.9mg**
Avocado (1 med)	**K 708mg, Mg 58mg, Cu 0.3mg**
Butternut squash	**K 582mg, Mg 59mg, Mn 0.5mg**
Sweet potato (1 med)	**K 542mg, Mg 31mg, Mn 0.5mg**
Broccoli (1 cup)	**K 457mg, Mg 33mg, Cr 22mcg**

Fruits

Food	Key Minerals
Dried apricots (½ cup)	K 755mg, Fe 1.9mg, Cu 0.2mg
Prunes (½ cup)	K 637mg, Mg 36mg, Fe 0.8mg
Raisins (½ cup)	K 543mg, Fe 1.4mg, Mn 0.1mg
Dried figs (½ cup)	K 507mg, Ca 121mg, Mg 50mg
Banana (1 med)	K 422mg, Mg 32mg, Mn 0.3mg

Grains

Food	Key Minerals
Quinoa (1 cup)	Mg 118mg, Fe 2.8mg, Mn 1.2mg
Brown rice (1 cup)	Mg 84mg, Mn 2.1mg, Se 19mcg
Oatmeal (1 cup)	Mg 63mg, Fe 2.1mg, Zn 1.1mg
Whole wheat pasta	Mg 42mg, Fe 1.5mg, Zn 1.1mg
Whole wheat bread	Mg 23mg, Se 10mcg, Mn 0.6mg

Meat & Poultry

Food	Key Minerals
Beef liver (3 oz)	Cu 12.4mg, Fe 5mg, Zn 5.3mg
Beef, lean (3 oz)	Zn 7mg, Fe 2.5mg, Se 33mcg
Pork tenderloin (3 oz)	Se 33mcg, Zn 2.9mg, K 356mg
Turkey breast (3 oz)	Se 27mcg, Zn 1.5mg, P 182mg
Chicken, dark (3 oz)	Zn 2.4mg, Fe 1.1mg, Se 18mcg

Vegetarian & Vegan Mineral Sources

Plant-based eaters face specific challenges. Here's your complete guide.

Iron for Vegetarians & Vegans

Plant iron (non-heme) absorbs at 5–12% compared to 15–35% for animal iron.
Solution: Pair with vitamin C and you'll absorb 2–3 times more.

Food	Serving	Iron
Fortified breakfast cereal	**1 serving**	**18 mg**
Lentils, cooked	**1 cup**	**6.6 mg**
Spinach, cooked	**1 cup**	**6.4 mg**
Blackstrap molasses	**1 Tbsp**	**3.5 mg**
Tofu, firm	**½ cup**	**3.4 mg**
Quinoa, cooked	**1 cup**	**2.8 mg**
Kidney beans, cooked	**½ cup**	**2.6 mg**
Tempeh	**½ cup**	**2.2 mg**

Iron + Vitamin C Pairings

Lentils + tomato sauce
Iron absorption ↑ 2–3x

Spinach + lemon juice
Citric acid enhances

Beans + salsa
Tomatoes = vitamin C

Tofu stir-fry + bell peppers
Peppers are C powerhouses

Oatmeal + strawberries
Berries boost uptake

Fortified cereal + OJ
Classic combo

Zinc for Vegetarians & Vegans

Plant zinc is bound by phytates in grains, beans, and seeds—reducing absorption by 50%. Soaking, sprouting, or fermenting reduces phytates.

Food	Serving	Zinc
Hemp seeds	**3 Tbsp**	**3.0 mg**
Chickpeas, cooked	**1 cup**	**2.5 mg**
Lentils, cooked	**1 cup**	**2.5 mg**
Oatmeal, cooked	**1 cup**	**2.3 mg**
Pumpkin seeds	**1 oz**	**2.2 mg**
Tofu, firm	**½ cup**	**2.0 mg**
Cashews	**1 oz**	**1.6 mg**
Tempeh	**½ cup**	**1.6 mg**

Pro Tip

Vegetarians may need 50% more zinc than meat-eaters. Consider 15–25 mg supplementation if eating mostly whole grains and legumes.

Calcium Without Dairy

You need 1,000–1,200 mg daily. Here's how to hit that without milk or cheese.

Food	Serving	Calcium
Fortified plant milk	**1 cup**	**300 mg**
Fortified orange juice	**1 cup**	**300 mg**
Collard greens, cooked	**1 cup**	**268 mg**
Calcium-set tofu	**½ cup**	**253 mg**
White beans, cooked	**1 cup**	**161 mg**
Bok choy, cooked	**1 cup**	**158 mg**
Tahini	**2 Tbsp**	**130 mg**
Kale, cooked	**1 cup**	**94 mg**
Almonds	**1 oz**	**76 mg**

Sample 1,000 mg Calcium Day

- **Breakfast:** Fortified plant milk on cereal (300 mg)
- **Lunch:** Tofu scramble (250 mg) + collard greens (135 mg)
- **Snack:** Almonds (76 mg)
- **Dinner:** Tahini dressing (65 mg) + white beans (160 mg)

= **986 mg** ✓

Magnesium (Easy to Get)

Food	Amount
Hemp seeds (3 Tbsp)	**210 mg**
Pumpkin seeds (1 oz)	**156 mg**
Spinach, cooked (1 cup)	**157 mg**
Black beans (1 cup)	**120 mg**
Chia seeds (1 oz)	**95 mg**
Almonds (1 oz)	**80 mg**

Iodine (Often Missed)

Food	Amount
Iodized salt (¼ tsp)	**71 mcg**
Seaweed/nori (1 sheet)	**16–43 mcg**
Navy beans (½ cup)	**32 mcg**
Prunes (5)	**13 mcg**

Note

If you avoid iodized salt and seaweed, consider a 150 mcg iodine supplement.

Budget-Friendly Mineral-Rich Foods

You don't need expensive superfoods. The best mineral sources are often the cheapest.

Best Mineral Value for Your Money

Food	What You Get	Key Minerals
Dried beans (any type)	1 lb = ~6 cups cooked	Fe, Mg, K, Zn
Dried lentils	1 lb = ~7 cups cooked	Fe, Mg, K, Zn
Eggs	1 dozen	Se, I, P, Zn
Frozen spinach	1 lb bag	Mg, K, Fe, Ca
Canned sardines	1 can (3.75 oz)	Ca, Se, P
Peanut butter	16 oz jar	Mg, K, Zn
Oats	Large canister	Mg, Fe, Zn, Mn
Bananas	1 lb (3–4 bananas)	K, Mg, Mn
Sweet potatoes	1 lb (2–3 medium)	K, Mn, Cu
Canned white beans	15 oz can	Fe, Mg, K

Budget Swaps for Expensive Foods

Expensive Option	→	Affordable Swap
Salmon	→	Canned sardines—Same Ca, more Se
Beef	→	Lentils—More Fe per serving, fraction of cost
Almonds	→	Peanuts—Similar Mg, much cheaper
Quinoa	→	Brown rice—Good Mg, Mn, Se at lower cost
Fresh spinach	→	Frozen spinach—Same minerals, lasts longer
Oysters	→	Pumpkin seeds—Good Zn alternative

Store Brand = Name Brand for

Canned beans (just rinse for sodium), frozen vegetables, dried grains and legumes, oats, eggs (shell color doesn't affect nutrition).

The Affordable Weekly Mineral Plan

Shopping List (All Budget-Friendly)	What This Covers
• **Dried black beans, 2 lbs** • **Brown rice, 2 lbs** • **Oats, large canister** • **Eggs, 1 dozen** • **Frozen spinach, 2 bags**	**Magnesium:** Oats, beans, spinach, peanut butter **Iron:** Beans, spinach, eggs, oats **Zinc:** Eggs, beans, oats, peanut butter **Potassium:** Beans, bananas, spinach, sweet potatoes
• **Bananas, 2 lbs** • **Peanut butter, 1 jar** • **Sweet potatoes, 2 lbs**	**Selenium:** Eggs, rice

Quick Mineral Boosters

Need to boost a specific mineral fast? Add these to any meal.

Add These to Any Meal

Add This	Mineral Boost	How to Use
Pumpkin seeds (1 Tbsp)	**Mg +39mg, Zn +0.6mg**	**Salads, oatmeal, yogurt**
Hemp seeds (1 Tbsp)	**Mg +70mg, Zn +1mg**	**Smoothies, salads, cereal**
Chia seeds (1 Tbsp)	**Mg +24mg, Ca +45mg**	**Yogurt, oatmeal, pudding**
Blackstrap molasses (1 tsp)	**Fe +1.2mg, Ca +41mg**	**Oatmeal, baked goods**
Nutritional yeast (2 Tbsp)	**Zn +3mg, Se +7mcg**	**Popcorn, pasta, eggs**
Dark chocolate chips (1 Tbsp)	**Mg +16mg, Fe +0.8mg**	**Trail mix, oatmeal**
Sunflower seeds (1 Tbsp)	**Se +6mcg, Mg +9mg**	**Salads, yogurt, stir-fries**
Tahini (1 Tbsp)	**Ca +64mg, Mg +14mg**	**Bowls, dressings**

5-Minute Mineral Snacks

Apple + 2 Tbsp peanut butter
K 350mg, Mg 50mg, Zn 0.9mg

Banana + pumpkin seeds
K 450mg, Mg 195mg, Zn 2.2mg

Yogurt + 1 oz almonds
Ca 490mg, Mg 117mg, Zn 1.3mg

Hummus + veggies
Fe 2mg, Mg 35mg, Zn 1.3mg

Trail mix (nuts + dark choc)
Mg 80mg, Fe 2mg, Zn 1.5mg

Cheese + whole grain crackers
Ca 200mg, Zn 1mg, Se 5mcg

Hard-boiled egg + toast
Se 15mcg, I 24mcg, Fe 1mg

Cottage cheese + fruit
Ca 138mg, Se 20mcg, P 358mg

One-Ingredient Upgrades

Simple swaps that boost minerals without changing your meals:

Swap This	→	For This
White rice	→	**Brown rice: +84mg Mg, +2mg Mn per cup**
White bread	→	**Whole wheat: +23mg Mg, +0.6mg Mn per slice**
Iceberg lettuce	→	**Spinach: +24mg Mg, +0.8mg Fe per cup**
Regular salt	→	**Iodized salt: +71mcg I per ¼ tsp**
Milk chocolate	→	**Dark chocolate: +40mg Mg, +2mg Fe per oz**
Potato chips	→	**Pumpkin seeds: +156mg Mg, +2.2mg Zn per oz**
Sour cream	→	**Greek yogurt: +200mg Ca, +200mg K per cup**
Mayo	→	**Tahini: +64mg Ca, +14mg Mg per Tbsp**

The 3-Foods-a-Day Method

If you eat these three foods every day, you'll cover most of your mineral bases:

1 serving dark leafy greens
Spinach, kale, or collards
= Mg, K, Fe, Ca

1 serving beans or lentils
Any type
= Fe, Mg, K, Zn

1 small handful seeds
Pumpkin, hemp, or chia
= Mg, Zn, Fe, Se

Add a variety of other whole foods around these three pillars, and you'll rarely need to worry about mineral deficiency.

Quick Reference: Daily Mineral Targets

How much do you need? Here's the quick summary:

Mineral	Daily Need	Top Sources
Magnesium	**310–420 mg**	**Pumpkin seeds, spinach, almonds, black beans**
Iron	**8–18 mg**	**Lentils, beef, fortified cereal, spinach**
Zinc	**8–11 mg**	**Oysters, beef, pumpkin seeds, chickpeas**
Calcium	**1000–1200 mg**	**Dairy, fortified foods, sardines, leafy greens**
Potassium	**2600–3400 mg**	**Potato, beans, banana, spinach, avocado**
Selenium	**55 mcg**	**Brazil nuts (1–2), seafood, eggs, turkey**
Iodine	**150 mcg**	**Iodized salt, seaweed, dairy, seafood**
Copper	**900 mcg**	**Liver, oysters, cashews, dark chocolate**
Chromium	**20–35 mcg**	**Broccoli, grape juice, whole grains**

Remember

Food first, supplements second. These charts give you everything you need to build a mineral-rich diet from whole foods.

APPENDIX D—MEDICATION-MINERAL DEPLETION CHART

Know what your medications deplete—and what to replace

Important

Many common medications deplete minerals from your body. This doesn't mean you should stop your medication—it means you should know what to replace. Always tell your doctor about supplements you're taking. Some supplements can interfere with how your medications work.

Organized by Medication Class

Find your medication below to see which minerals it may deplete

Acid-Blocking Medications

PPIs and H2 blockers reduce stomach acid, which is needed to absorb many minerals.

Proton Pump Inhibitors (PPIs)

Prilosec (omeprazole), Nexium (esomeprazole), Prevacid (lansoprazole), Protonix (pantoprazole), Aciphex (rabeprazole), Dexilant

Minerals Depleted	What to Do
Magnesium	**Supplement 200–400 mg Mg glycinate daily**
Calcium	**Take calcium citrate (not carbonate) with food**
Iron	**Take iron on empty stomach, 2 hrs apart from PPI**
Zinc	**Consider 15–25 mg zinc if on long-term PPI**
Vitamin B12	**Supplement B12 (not a mineral but commonly depleted)**

Why this happens

Stomach acid is required to release minerals from food and convert them to absorbable forms. Less acid = less mineral absorption.

H2 Blockers

Pepcid (famotidine), Tagamet (cimetidine)

Mineral Depleted	What to Do
Calcium, Iron, Zinc	**Same as PPIs but less severe**
Zinc (Tagamet especially)	**Supplement 15–25 mg zinc daily**

Antacids

Tums (calcium carbonate), Maalox, Mylanta, Rolaids, Gaviscon, Milk of Magnesia

Mineral Depleted	What to Do
Iron	**Take iron 2+ hours apart from antacids**
Zinc	**Consider 15–25 mg zinc if using antacids regularly**
Phosphorus	**Usually not a concern with occasional use**
Magnesium (aluminum-containing)	**Aluminum antacids can deplete magnesium**

> **Note**
>
> Tums contains calcium, so it won't deplete calcium—but it neutralizes stomach acid needed to absorb calcium from food. Calcium carbonate in Tums is poorly absorbed without stomach acid. If using Tums regularly, you may still need a calcium citrate supplement.

Blood Pressure Medications

Loop Diuretics

Lasix (furosemide), Bumex (bumetanide), Edecrin (ethacrynic acid)

Mineral Depleted	What to Do
Potassium	**Eat potassium-rich foods; may need Rx supplement**
Magnesium	**Supplement 200–400 mg Mg daily**
Calcium	**Supplement 500–1000 mg calcium citrate**
Zinc	**Consider 15–25 mg zinc daily**

Thiazide Diuretics

Hydrochlorothiazide (HCTZ), Chlorthalidone, Microzide, Diuril

Mineral Depleted	What to Do
Potassium	**Eat potassium-rich foods; may need Rx supplement**
Magnesium	**Supplement 200–400 mg Mg daily**
Zinc	**Consider 15–25 mg zinc daily**

> **Note**
>
> Thiazides actually INCREASE calcium retention (good for bones), unlike loop diuretics.

Potassium-Sparing Diuretics

Aldactone (spironolactone), Inspra (eplerenone), Dyrenium (triamterene), Midamor (amiloride)

> **WARNING**
>
> **Never take potassium supplements with potassium-sparing diuretics. This can cause life-threatening heart rhythms. These medications preserve potassium—do NOT supplement!**

ACE Inhibitors

Lisinopril, Enalapril, Benazepril, Ramipril, Captopril

Mineral Affected	What to Do
Zinc (depleted)	**Consider 15–25 mg zinc daily**
Potassium (INCREASES)	**Do NOT supplement potassium without testing**

ARBs (Angiotensin Receptor Blockers)

Losartan, Valsartan, Irbesartan, Olmesartan

Mineral Affected	What to Do
Zinc (possible)	**Consider 15–25 mg zinc if symptomatic**
Potassium (INCREASES)	**Do NOT supplement potassium without testing**

Diabetes Medications

Metformin

Glucophage, Glumetza, Fortamet, Riomet

Nutrient Depleted	What to Do
Vitamin B12	**Supplement B12 500–1000 mcg daily (critical)**
Magnesium (possible)	**Consider 200–300 mg Mg if symptomatic**
Zinc (possible)	**Consider 15 mg zinc daily**

> **Note**
>
> Metformin is one of the safest diabetes drugs, but long-term use requires B12 monitoring. Ask for annual B12 testing.

SGLT2 Inhibitors

Jardiance (empagliflozin), Farxiga (dapagliflozin), Invokana (canagliflozin), Steglatro (ertugliflozin)

Mineral Depleted	What to Do
Magnesium	**Consider 200–300 mg Mg glycinate daily**
Potassium	**Monitor levels; eat potassium-rich foods**
Phosphorus	**Usually resolves; monitor if symptomatic**

> **Note**
>
> SGLT2 inhibitors increase urination, which can flush out minerals. These medications are increasingly prescribed for heart failure as well as diabetes. If you take both metformin and an SGLT2 inhibitor, mineral monitoring becomes even more important.

Cholesterol Medications

Statins

Lipitor (atorvastatin), Crestor (rosuvastatin), Zocor (simvastatin), Pravachol (pravastatin)

Nutrient Depleted	What to Do
CoQ10 (not a mineral)	**Supplement CoQ10 100–200 mg daily**
Selenium (possible)	**Consider 50–100 mcg selenium if symptomatic**

Bile Acid Sequestrants

Questran (cholestyramine), Welchol (colesevelam), Colestid (colestipol)

Mineral Depleted	What to Do
Iron, Zinc, Calcium, Magnesium	**Take ALL minerals 4–6 hours apart from medication**

> **Why**
>
> These medications bind minerals in the gut and prevent absorption.

Osteoporosis Medications

Bisphosphonates

Fosamax (alendronate), Boniva (ibandronate), Actonel (risedronate), Reclast (zoledronic acid)

Mineral Affected	What to Do
Calcium (blocks absorption)	**Take calcium 2+ hours AFTER medication**
Magnesium (blocks absorption)	**Take magnesium 2+ hours AFTER medication**
Iron (blocks absorption)	**Take iron 2+ hours AFTER medication**

> **Critical**
>
> **Take bisphosphonates on an empty stomach with plain water only. Wait 30–60 minutes before eating, drinking anything else, or taking any supplements.**

Antibiotics

Fluoroquinolones

Cipro (ciprofloxacin), Levaquin (levofloxacin), Avelox (moxifloxacin)

Minerals Affected	What to Do
Magnesium, Calcium, Iron, Zinc	**Take ALL minerals 2+ hours apart from antibiotic**

> **Why**
>
> These minerals bind to fluoroquinolones and make BOTH less effective.

Tetracyclines

Doxycycline, Minocycline, Tetracycline

Minerals Affected	What to Do
Calcium, Magnesium, Iron, Zinc	**Take ALL minerals 2+ hours apart from antibiotic**

NSAIDs (Pain Relievers)

Ibuprofen (Advil, Motrin), Naproxen (Aleve), Aspirin, Indomethacin (Indocin), Meloxicam (Mobic), Celecoxib (Celebrex)

Mineral Depleted	What to Do
Magnesium	**Consider 200–300 mg Mg glycinate daily**
Potassium	**Eat potassium-rich foods; monitor if on long-term use**
Zinc	**Consider 15–25 mg zinc if using NSAIDs regularly**
Calcium	**Ensure adequate calcium intake**

Why

NSAIDs can damage the gut lining, reducing mineral absorption. Long-term use also increases urinary excretion of some minerals and may affect kidney handling of electrolytes.

Note

Occasional NSAID use (a few days for acute pain) is unlikely to cause significant mineral depletion. The concern is with regular, long-term use for chronic conditions like arthritis.

Corticosteroids

Prednisone, Prednisolone, Dexamethasone, Methylprednisolone, Hydrocortisone

Mineral Depleted	What to Do
Calcium	**Supplement 1000–1200 mg calcium daily**
Potassium	**Eat potassium-rich foods daily**
Magnesium	**Supplement 200–400 mg Mg daily**
Zinc	**Consider 15–25 mg zinc daily**
Chromium	**Consider 200 mcg chromium (helps blood sugar)**

Critical

Long-term corticosteroid use causes significant bone loss. Calcium, vitamin D, magnesium, and vitamin K2 are essential. Consider a bone density test.

Hormone Medications

Birth Control Pills & HRT

Oral contraceptives, estrogen replacement therapy, hormone replacement therapy

Mineral Affected	What to Do
Magnesium	**Consider 200–300 mg Mg daily**
Zinc	**Consider 15 mg zinc daily**
Copper (INCREASES)	**Usually not a problem unless already high**

Seizure Medications (Anticonvulsants)

Dilantin (phenytoin), Tegretol (carbamazepine), Depakote (valproic acid), Phenobarbital

Mineral Depleted	What to Do
Calcium	**Supplement 1000 mg calcium daily**
Magnesium	**Supplement 200–400 mg Mg daily**
Zinc	**Consider 15–25 mg zinc daily**
Selenium	**Consider 50–100 mcg selenium**

Note

These medications increase bone loss risk. Calcium, vitamin D, and vitamin K are particularly important.

Lithium

Lithobid, Eskalith

Critical

Lithium levels are affected by sodium intake. Maintain consistent sodium intake—don't suddenly increase or decrease salt. Monitor thyroid function (iodine-related).

Organized by Mineral Depleted

Looking for all medications that deplete a specific mineral?

Magnesium

Medication Class	Examples
Proton pump inhibitors (PPIs)	**Prilosec, Nexium, Prevacid, Protonix**
Loop diuretics	**Lasix (furosemide), Bumex**
Thiazide diuretics	**HCTZ, Chlorthalidone**
SGLT2 inhibitors	**Jardiance, Farxiga, Invokana**
NSAIDs (long-term use)	**Ibuprofen, Naproxen, Aspirin**
Fluoroquinolone antibiotics	**Cipro, Levaquin (bind Mg)**
Tetracycline antibiotics	**Doxycycline, Minocycline (bind Mg)**
Corticosteroids	**Prednisone, Dexamethasone**
Estrogen-containing medications	**Birth control pills, HRT**
Aluminum-containing antacids	**Maalox, Mylanta**
Bisphosphonates	**Fosamax, Boniva (block absorption)**

What to do

Supplement 200–400 mg magnesium glycinate daily. Take 2+ hours apart from medications that bind magnesium.

Potassium

Medication Class	Examples
Loop diuretics	**Lasix (furosemide), Bumex—major depletion**
Thiazide diuretics	**HCTZ, Chlorthalidone—significant**
SGLT2 inhibitors	**Jardiance, Farxiga, Invokana**
Corticosteroids	**Prednisone, Dexamethasone**
NSAIDs (long-term use)	**Ibuprofen, Naproxen, Aspirin**
Stimulant laxatives (long-term)	**Dulcolax, Senokot**
Some asthma medications	**Albuterol, Salmeterol (high doses)**

What to do

Eat potassium-rich foods (potatoes, bananas, beans, leafy greens). Do NOT take potassium supplements without a doctor's order—excess potassium is dangerous.

WARNING

Some medications INCREASE potassium (ACE inhibitors, ARBs, potassium-sparing diuretics). Never supplement potassium if you take these medications.

Calcium

Medication Class	Examples
Proton pump inhibitors (PPIs)	**Prilosec, Nexium, Prevacid**
Loop diuretics	**Lasix, Bumex**
Corticosteroids	**Prednisone, Dexamethasone—major effect**
Anticonvulsants	**Dilantin, Tegretol, Phenobarbital**
NSAIDs (long-term use)	**Ibuprofen, Naproxen, Aspirin**
Antacids (reduce absorption)	**Tums, Maalox (neutralize stomach acid)**
Fluoroquinolone/Tetracycline antibiotics	**Cipro, Doxycycline (bind calcium)**

Bisphosphonates	**Fosamax, Boniva (block absorption)**
Thyroid medications	**Synthroid, Levoxyl (bind calcium)**
Bile acid sequestrants	**Questran, Welchol**

What to do

Supplement calcium citrate (better absorbed with low stomach acid). Take 2+ hours apart from medications that bind calcium.

Note: Thiazide diuretics actually INCREASE calcium retention and may protect bones.

Zinc

Medication Class	Examples
Proton pump inhibitors (PPIs)	**Prilosec, Nexium, Prevacid**
H2 blockers	**Tagamet (especially), Pepcid**
Antacids	**Tums, Maalox, Rolaids**
ACE inhibitors	**Lisinopril, Enalapril**
Loop and Thiazide diuretics	**Lasix, HCTZ, Chlorthalidone**
NSAIDs (long-term use)	**Ibuprofen, Naproxen, Aspirin**
Corticosteroids	**Prednisone, Dexamethasone**
Estrogen-containing medications	**Birth control pills, HRT**
Fluoroquinolone/Tetracycline antibiotics	**Cipro, Doxycycline (bind zinc)**
Penicillamine	**Used for Wilson's disease, RA**

What to do

Supplement 15–25 mg zinc picolinate or citrate daily. Take 2+ hours apart from antibiotics that bind zinc.

Iron

Medication Class	Examples
Proton pump inhibitors (PPIs)	**Prilosec, Nexium—reduce stomach acid**
H2 blockers	**Pepcid, Tagamet—reduce stomach acid**
Antacids	**Tums, Maalox—neutralize stomach acid**
Fluoroquinolone/Tetracycline antibiotics	**Cipro, Doxycycline (bind iron)**
Bisphosphonates	**Fosamax, Boniva (bind iron)**
Bile acid sequestrants	**Questran, Welchol (bind iron)**
Thyroid medications	**Synthroid (bind iron)**

What to do

Take iron on empty stomach with vitamin C for absorption. Take 2–4+ hours apart from medications that bind or reduce iron absorption.

Test before supplementing—excess iron is toxic.

Selenium

Medication Class	Examples
Corticosteroids	**Prednisone, Dexamethasone**
Anticonvulsants	**Dilantin, Tegretol, Valproic acid**
Statins (possible)	**Lipitor, Crestor (research mixed)**

What to do

Consider 50–100 mcg selenium daily if on long-term therapy. Don't exceed 200 mcg without medical supervision.

Quick Reference

Common medication situations and what to supplement

If You Take a PPI Daily (Prilosec, Nexium, etc.)

- **Magnesium glycinate:** 200–400 mg daily
- **Calcium citrate:** 500–1000 mg daily (split doses)
- **Vitamin B12:** 500–1000 mcg daily
- **Consider:** Zinc 15 mg daily

Timing: Take supplements 2+ hours apart from PPI for best absorption.

If You Take a Loop or Thiazide Diuretic

- **Magnesium glycinate:** 200–400 mg daily
- **Potassium:** Eat potassium-rich foods (may need Rx supplement)
- **Zinc:** 15–25 mg daily
- **For loop diuretics only:** Calcium citrate 500–1000 mg daily

Monitoring: Ask your doctor about regular electrolyte checks.

If You Take Corticosteroids Long-Term

- **Calcium citrate:** 1000–1200 mg daily (split doses)
- **Vitamin D:** 2000–4000 IU daily
- **Magnesium glycinate:** 200–400 mg daily
- **Zinc:** 15–25 mg daily
- **Potassium:** Eat potassium-rich foods daily
- **Chromium:** 200 mcg daily (helps blood sugar)

Critical: Bone loss is a major concern. Consider a bone density test.

If You Take Metformin

- **Vitamin B12:** 500–1000 mcg daily (critical)
- **Consider:** Magnesium 200–300 mg daily
- **Consider:** Zinc 15 mg daily

Monitoring: Ask for annual B12 level testing if on long-term metformin.

If You Take an Antibiotic Course (Cipro, Doxycycline, etc.)

- Continue your regular mineral supplements
- Take ALL minerals **2+ hours apart** from antibiotic doses
- Don't take calcium, magnesium, zinc, or iron with the antibiotic pill

Why: These minerals bind to certain antibiotics and make both less effective.

If You Take NSAIDs Regularly (Ibuprofen, Naproxen, Aspirin)

- **Magnesium glycinate:** 200–300 mg daily
- **Zinc:** 15–25 mg daily
- **Potassium:** Eat potassium-rich foods daily
- **Consider:** Calcium if intake is low

Note: Occasional use for acute pain is unlikely to cause significant depletion. This applies to daily or near-daily use for chronic conditions.

Timing Your Supplements Around Medications

Medication	When to Take Minerals
Thyroid medication (Synthroid)	Take minerals 4+ hours AFTER thyroid med
Bisphosphonates (Fosamax)	Take minerals 2+ hours AFTER bisphosphonate
Fluoroquinolones (Cipro)	Take minerals 2+ hours BEFORE or 6 hours AFTER
Tetracyclines (Doxycycline)	Take minerals 2+ hours BEFORE or 4 hours AFTER
PPIs (Prilosec)	Take minerals with food, 2+ hours from PPI
Iron supplements	Take 2 hours apart from most other medications

When to Talk to Your Doctor

- **Before starting any new supplement if you're on prescription medications**
- **If you take blood thinners (warfarin, etc.)**
- **If you have kidney disease (affects potassium, magnesium handling)**
- **If you take potassium-sparing diuretics or ACE inhibitors/ARBs**
- **If you're on multiple medications that deplete the same mineral**
- **If you experience new symptoms after starting a supplement**

The charts in this appendix are based on documented drug-nutrient interactions. However, individual responses vary. When in doubt, ask your pharmacist or doctor.

Know what your medications deplete—and what to replace

APPENDIX E—LAB TEST QUICK REFERENCE

"Normal" doesn't always mean "optimal"

Lab reference ranges are based on population averages—which includes a lot of people who don't feel great. This quick reference shows both standard ranges and the narrower **optimal ranges** where most people feel their best.

Key Mineral Tests

Test	Standard Range	Optimal Range	Notes
Ferritin (iron stores)	12–150 ng/mL (women) 12–300 ng/mL (men)	**50–100 ng/mL**	Below 30 = low; test before supplementing iron. Target varies by condition—see relevant chapter.
Serum Iron	60–170 mcg/dL	**Mid-range**	Less useful alone; pair with ferritin & TIBC.
RBC Magnesium	4.2–6.8 mg/dL	**5.5–6.5 mg/dL**	Better than serum Mg (blood level often normal when deficient).
Serum Magnesium	1.7–2.2 mg/dL	**2.0–2.2 mg/dL**	Only 1% of body Mg is in blood; can miss deficiency.
Zinc (plasma/serum)	60–120 mcg/dL	**80–120 mcg/dL**	Fasting morning sample most accurate.
Selenium (serum)	70–150 ng/mL	**100–130 ng/mL**	Above 200 = excess risk.
TSH (thyroid)	0.4–4.5 mIU/L	**1.0–2.5 mIU/L**	Reflects iodine status indirectly.
Potassium (serum)	3.5–5.0 mEq/L	**4.0–4.5 mEq/L**	Narrow range; both low and high are dangerous.
Sodium (serum)	136–145 mEq/L	**Mid-range**	Rarely deficient from diet.

What Tests to Request

If you suspect mineral deficiency, ask for these:

- Iron panel: Ferritin, serum iron, TIBC, transferrin saturation (not just CBC)
- Magnesium: RBC magnesium if available (more accurate than serum)
- Thyroid: TSH, Free T4, Free T3 (reflects iodine and selenium status)
- Zinc and selenium: Serum levels (fasting morning draw)
- Vitamin D: 25-hydroxyvitamin D (affects calcium absorption)

Three Things to Know

1. **"Normal" is not "optimal."** You can be at the low end of normal and still have symptoms. Many practitioners aim for mid-range or optimal values.

2. **Ranges vary by lab.** Always compare your results to the reference range printed on YOUR lab report—different labs use slightly different ranges.

3. **One test isn't the whole picture.** Symptoms matter. If your levels are "normal" but you have classic deficiency symptoms, discuss this with your doctor.

> **Self-Advocacy Tip**
>
> If your doctor dismisses your concerns because your labs are "normal," you can say:
>
> ***"I understand it's in the reference range, but I'm at the low end and still having symptoms. Can we discuss whether optimizing this level might help?"***

Your labs. Your body. Your voice.

GLOSSARY

Your Labs Are Fine. You're Not.

How to Use This Glossary

This glossary provides definitions for key terms, concepts, and frameworks used throughout the book. Terms are organized alphabetically for easy reference.

You'll find several types of entries:

A

3 AM Wake-Up Pattern

A sleep disturbance characterized by waking after 4–5 hours of sleep, fully alert, unable to return to sleep. Usually indicates cortisol spiking when it should be at its lowest point, often related to magnesium deficiency or blood sugar crashes.

80/20 Rule (for mineral health)

The principle that 20% of actions produce 80% of results. High-impact 20%: paying attention to body signals, addressing deficiencies that clearly affect your life, maintaining food sources, monitoring high-risk situations, and periodic retesting. Low-impact 80%: perfect timing, perfect daily consistency, taking every mineral "just in case," obsessive tracking, and constant testing.

Absolute Minimum Protocol

A streamlined intervention for readers in Protection mode, consisting of three foods (spinach, canned black beans, pumpkin seeds) plus magnesium glycinate 200 mg at bedtime. Designed to provide essential mineral support with minimal effort for those who are barely functioning.

Absorption Blockers

Substances that interfere with mineral absorption when taken together. Calcium and iron compete for absorption. Coffee and tea block iron. Calcium interferes with thyroid medication. Proper timing (separating by 2–4 hours) prevents these interactions.

ACE Inhibitors

Blood pressure medications with names ending in "-pril" (such as lisinopril and enalapril) that deplete zinc. Readers taking these medications should consider zinc testing and supplementation.

ACEs Study (Adverse Childhood Experiences Study)

Landmark research studying over 17,000 people that demonstrated childhood trauma significantly affects adult health for decades, including higher rates of heart disease, diabetes, autoimmune conditions, and chronic inflammation. Explains why some people have chronically dysregulated nervous systems.

Army Framework

A conceptual model for understanding immune function. Zinc serves as the commander (develops and coordinates immune cells), selenium as the armor (protects immune cells from oxidative damage), vitamin D as the intelligence (activates defenses and coordinates response), and iron as the supply line (supports rapid immune cell deployment).

B

Bariatric Surgery

Weight loss surgeries such as gastric bypass or sleeve gastrectomy that permanently alter nutrient absorption. Mineral testing is mandatory for anyone who has had these procedures.

B-Complex

A supplement containing the eight B vitamins. Best taken in the morning due to energizing effects. Particularly important for vegetarians, people over 50, and those taking metformin.

Benign PVCs (Premature Ventricular Contractions)

Extra heartbeats originating in the ventricles that feel like fluttering, skipped beats, or pounding. Often dismissed by cardiologists but frequently related to magnesium deficiency.

C

Calcium Carbonate

A form of calcium supplement that requires stomach acid for absorption and should be taken with food. Less ideal than calcium citrate for people with low stomach acid.

Calcium Citrate

A form of calcium supplement that absorbs without stomach acid and can be taken at any time. Preferred over calcium carbonate for people with low stomach acid or those over 65.

Calcium-Set Tofu

Tofu made using calcium sulfate as a coagulant, resulting in significantly higher calcium content than other tofu varieties. A key protein and calcium source for vegetarians.

Carbonyl Iron

A gentle, well-absorbed form of supplemental iron that causes fewer gastrointestinal side effects than ferrous sulfate.

CBT-I (Cognitive Behavioral Therapy for Insomnia)

A highly effective therapeutic approach for chronic insomnia, often more effective than medication. Addresses thoughts and behaviors that perpetuate sleep problems.

Cold and Flu Season

Reframed in the book as "vitamin D deficiency season." During winter months in northern latitudes, skin cannot make vitamin D from sun exposure, leading to population-wide deficiency and weakened respiratory defenses.

Complete Iron Panel

A set of three blood tests that together provide a complete picture of iron status: ferritin (iron stores), serum iron (circulating iron), and TIBC (iron transport capacity). More informative than any single iron test.

ConsumerLab.com Approved

A third-party testing seal indicating that a supplement has been independently verified for contents, purity, and quality.

Corticosteroids

Anti-inflammatory medications such as prednisone that deplete calcium, potassium, and magnesium. Long-term users should monitor mineral levels.

Cortisol

A stress hormone released by the adrenal glands during the fight-or-flight response. Chronically elevated cortisol depletes magnesium, disrupts sleep, impairs digestion, and accelerates mineral depletion. Should be highest in the morning and lowest around midnight.

D

DASH Diet (Dietary Approaches to Stop Hypertension)

An eating pattern proven to lower blood pressure by 8–14 mmHg, comparable to medication. Works primarily by dramatically increasing potassium, magnesium, and calcium while moderating sodium.

DEXA Scan

A bone density scan that measures bone mineral density. Recommended for baseline assessment in menopausal women to track bone health.

Diffuse Thinning

A pattern of hair loss characterized by overall thinning rather than bald patches. Often indicates systemic deficiency, particularly iron.

Digoxin

A heart medication that becomes toxic if magnesium or potassium levels drop too low. Mineral testing is mandatory for anyone taking this medication.

Direct-to-Consumer Testing

Laboratory testing ordered by individuals without requiring a doctor's prescription. Services include Quest Direct, Labcorp OnDemand, Ulta Lab Tests, and Walk-In Lab. Typically costs $50–150 per test. An option when doctors won't order requested tests.

Diuretics

Medications (also called "water pills") such as HCTZ, Lasix, and Chlorthalidone that actively drain potassium, magnesium, and zinc from the body. Long-term users require mineral testing and likely supplementation.

Dopamine

A neurotransmitter responsible for motivation, pleasure, focus, and movement control. The enzyme that produces dopamine requires iron. Low iron leads to low dopamine, causing symptoms that mimic depression.

Double Whammy

The combination of declining peptide production (due to age) and chronic nervous system dysregulation (due to stress), which together prevent the body from properly utilizing minerals even when intake is adequate. Common in people over 40 who are chronically stressed.

E

Elemental Iron

The actual amount of absorbable iron in a supplement, as opposed to the total weight of the iron compound. The number to look for on supplement labels when determining dose.

Emotional Acceptance

The practice of being present with emotions without judgment, as opposed to experiential avoidance. Research shows emotional acceptance decreases stress and supports nervous system regulation.

Every-Other-Day Dosing

A dosing strategy particularly useful for iron, where research shows absorption may actually be better with alternate-day dosing rather than daily. Also reduces side effects like constipation and nausea.

Experiential Avoidance

Actively trying to avoid or suppress inner emotional experiences. Research shows this increases stress, anxiety, and nervous system dysregulation rather than reducing it.

F

Falling Off

The common experience of stopping a supplement routine due to forgetting, life circumstances, or loss of motivation. Reframed in the book as normal human behavior rather than moral failure.

Feel-Pause-Act

The book's central framework for nervous system regulation. Feel: notice sensations and emotions without judgment. Pause: create space between feeling and reacting (often 60–90 seconds). Act: choose a response from awareness rather than automatic reaction. Based on research showing emotions peak and subside within 90 seconds when allowed without resistance.

Ferritin

A protein that stores iron in the body. Blood ferritin levels indicate iron reserves. Optimal levels: above 50 ng/mL for energy, above 70 ng/mL for hair health, above 75 ng/mL for Restless Legs Syndrome. Lab "normal" starts at 15, but many people feel terrible until levels are much higher.

Ferrous Bisglycinate

A chelated form of iron supplement that is gentle on the stomach and well-absorbed. Preferred over ferrous sulfate for better tolerability.

Ferrous Sulfate

A common but harsh form of iron supplement that often causes stomach upset and constipation. Effective but less tolerable than gentler forms.

Fight-or-Flight Mode (Gas Pedal)

The sympathetic nervous system response that prepares the body for action or danger. Increases heart rate, pumps blood to muscles, releases stress hormones, and sharpens focus on threats. Problematic when chronically activated, as it impairs digestion and accelerates mineral depletion.

Food First

The foundational principle that mineral-rich foods should be the primary source of nutrients, with supplements used to correct deficiencies rather than replace good eating habits. Does not mean "food only" or "perfect eating."

Four-to-Five Days Per Week

A realistic consistency target that is often sufficient for maintaining mineral status. Presented as an alternative to the perfectionist expectation of daily supplementation.

Free T3

The active form of thyroid hormone. T4 (inactive) must convert to T3 to function. Conversion requires selenium and zinc. You can have "normal" TSH but low Free T3 if conversion is impaired.

Functional Deficiency

A state in which mineral levels fall in the bottom third of the laboratory reference range and symptoms are present, even though the lab report shows results as "normal." Indicates suboptimal levels that cause symptoms without reaching the threshold for medical diagnosis.

G

GABA (Gamma-Aminobutyric Acid)

The brain's primary calming neurotransmitter. Quiets racing thoughts and reduces anxiety. Magnesium is required for GABA to function properly.

Grounding

A technique for returning to the present moment when numb or disconnected, using the five senses: name 5 things you can see, 4 you can touch, 3 you can hear, 2 you can smell, 1 you can taste.

Gut Lining

A single layer of cells separating the digestive tract from the bloodstream. Decides what gets absorbed and what stays out. When damaged, tight junctions become loose, allowing substances that shouldn't enter the bloodstream to pass through.

H

H. pylori (Helicobacter pylori)

A bacteria that infects the stomach, reduces stomach acid production, and impairs mineral absorption. Can contribute to persistent digestive symptoms.

Hashimoto's Thyroiditis

An autoimmune condition in which the immune system attacks the thyroid. Selenium supplementation (200 mcg daily) has been shown to reduce thyroid antibodies and may slow disease progression.

Healing Mode

A nervous system state characterized by engagement, curiosity, and capacity for strategic action and comprehensive change. In this state, the body can effectively absorb and utilize nutrients. Represented by the healing icon () in the book's check-ins.

Heme Iron

Iron found in animal foods (meat, poultry, fish) that absorbs approximately three times better than non-heme iron from plants.

Hepcidin

A peptide that regulates iron absorption from food and release from storage. An example of how peptide signaling directs mineral utilization.

High-Risk Times

Predictable periods when mineral needs increase or depletion accelerates: winter (vitamin D), menstruation (iron), high stress (magnesium), illness, travel. Proactively increasing support during these times prevents symptom return.

Hydrochloric Acid

Stomach acid that kills harmful bacteria, breaks down protein, and releases minerals from food so they can be absorbed. Many people, especially as they age, don't produce enough.

I

Increased Intestinal Permeability

A condition in which the gut lining barrier becomes more porous than it should be, allowing substances that shouldn't enter the bloodstream to pass through. Triggers inflammation and further impairs mineral absorption.

Informed-Choice

A third-party testing certification specifically designed for athletes, indicating that a supplement has been tested for banned substances and quality.

L

L-Glutamine

An amino acid that serves as the primary fuel for gut lining cells. Used to support gut lining repair. Typical dose: 5–10 grams daily.

Loop Diuretics

Blood pressure medications such as furosemide (Lasix) that deplete potassium, magnesium, and calcium. Patients should have mineral levels monitored and likely supplemented.

M

Magnificent Seven Foods

Seven food categories that cover approximately 90% of mineral needs when eaten weekly: (1) dark leafy greens, (2) beans and lentils, (3) nuts and seeds, (4) whole grains, (5) potatoes with skin, (6) yogurt and dairy (or fortified alternatives), and (7) meat, fish, or protein alternatives.

Magnesium Glycinate

A chelated form of magnesium bound to the amino acid glycine. Well-absorbed, calming, and unlikely to cause digestive upset. The preferred form for supplementation, especially when taken at bedtime.

Magnesium Oxide

A poorly absorbed, inexpensive form of magnesium often found in cheap supplements. Not recommended due to low bioavailability. Can cause diarrhea because unabsorbed magnesium pulls water into the intestines.

Maintenance Dose

The amount of a supplement needed to maintain adequate levels after a deficiency has been corrected. Typically 25–50% lower than the treatment dose. Found by gradually reducing the treatment dose until the minimum effective amount is identified.

Medication-Induced Depletion

Mineral losses caused by pharmaceutical drugs. PPIs deplete magnesium, calcium, iron, and B12. Diuretics deplete magnesium, potassium, and zinc. Metformin depletes B12. Birth control may deplete magnesium, zinc, and selenium. Requires proactive replacement rather than stopping medication.

Metformin

A diabetes medication that depletes B12 and possibly magnesium. Long-term users should monitor these nutrients and consider supplementation.

Mg-ATP

The functional form of ATP (the body's energy currency), which requires magnesium to be bound to it. Without adequate magnesium, cells cannot access energy even if ATP is present.

Minimum Effective Dose

The lowest amount of a supplement that keeps symptoms away. Found by reducing the dose that made you feel better by 25–50% after 2–3 months of consistent improvement, then monitoring for symptom return.

Muscle Switch

A conceptual model explaining muscle function: calcium turns muscles ON (contraction), magnesium turns them OFF (relaxation), and potassium regulates the electrical signals. Applies to skeletal muscles, heart muscle, blood vessel walls, and even the brain's ability to shift from alert to calm states.

N

Nervous System Hijacking

The phenomenon in which a minor setback (such as supplement side effects) triggers a disproportionate emotional response ("Nothing ever works for me, I should just give up"). Recognizing this pattern is essential for effective troubleshooting.

Neurotransmitter Factory

A conceptual model for understanding brain chemistry. The brain produces neurotransmitters from mineral raw materials: iron for dopamine, magnesium for GABA, zinc for serotonin. When raw materials run low, production suffers.

Non-Heme Iron

Iron found in plant foods (beans, spinach, fortified grains) that absorbs less efficiently than heme iron. Absorption improves significantly when paired with vitamin C.

Normal Labs, Terrible Symptoms

A common situation in which standard laboratory tests return within reference ranges but the person continues to experience significant symptoms. Causes include: wrong tests ordered, "normal" ranges being too broad, symptoms not caused by mineral deficiency, or multiple issues occurring simultaneously.

NSAIDs

Non-steroidal anti-inflammatory drugs such as Advil, Aleve, ibuprofen, and naproxen. Daily use can cause slow iron loss through gastrointestinal bleeding and can damage the gut lining.

NSF Certified

A third-party testing certification indicating that a supplement has been independently verified for contents, purity, and quality.

P

Peptides

Short chains of amino acids that carry specific messages throughout the body, telling minerals where to go and what to do. Production declines with age, particularly after the 30s, which can make minerals less efficient even when levels are adequate.

Performance Machine

A conceptual model for understanding athletic function. Iron delivers fuel (oxygen), magnesium powers the battery (ATP production), and electrolytes run the electrical system (muscle signals).

Permission to Quit

The book's acknowledgment that stopping supplementation is sometimes the right choice—not failure, but an active decision. Appropriate when interventions haven't helped after 4–6 months, when the pursuit of wellness creates more stress than the symptoms, when costs outweigh benefits, or when other priorities take precedence.

PMDD (Premenstrual Dysphoric Disorder)

A severe, disabling form of PMS causing significant mood symptoms in the week before menstruation. Requires comprehensive holistic treatment including nervous system regulation, signaling support, gut health, and mineral optimization.

Power Bowl

A meal formula consisting of a grain base, protein, vegetables, crunchy toppings, and dressing. Takes approximately 10 minutes to prepare and provides substantial mineral content.

Power Foods

Exceptionally mineral-dense foods deserving special attention: oysters (zinc), pumpkin seeds (magnesium, zinc), dark chocolate 70%+ (magnesium, iron), sardines with bones (calcium), Brazil nuts (selenium), and black strap molasses (iron, calcium, magnesium, potassium).

PPIs (Proton Pump Inhibitors)

Medications such as Prilosec, Nexium, Prevacid, and Protonix that reduce stomach acid. Long-term use (more than one year) blocks absorption of magnesium, iron, calcium, and B12. Testing is mandatory for long-term users.

Prebiotics

Foods that feed beneficial gut bacteria. Include garlic, onions, asparagus, slightly green bananas, and cooked and cooled potatoes or rice.

Probiotics

Beneficial bacteria that support digestion, mineral absorption, and gut lining health. Found in fermented foods (sauerkraut, kimchi, kefir) or supplements. Look for multi-strain formulas with at least 10–50 billion CFUs.

Protection Mode

A survival-oriented nervous system state characterized by overwhelm, shutdown, or fight-or-flight activation. In this state, the body cannot properly absorb or utilize nutrients due to reduced digestive blood flow, accelerated mineral depletion, increased inflammation, and disrupted peptide signaling. Represented by the protection icon ( ) in the book's check-ins.

R

RBC Magnesium (Red Blood Cell Magnesium)

A blood test measuring magnesium inside red blood cells, providing a more accurate picture of magnesium status than standard serum magnesium tests. The test to request specifically. Optimal placement is in the middle to top third of the reference range.

Reference Range

The range of values a laboratory considers "normal" for a given test, based on population averages. Being within range does not necessarily indicate optimal health; the Rule of Thirds provides more nuanced interpretation.

Regulated First, Optimized Second

The book's core principle that nervous system regulation takes priority over mineral optimization. When regulated, you hear body signals clearly, troubleshoot without panicking, and can be flexible. When dysregulated, every symptom feels like crisis and you can't tell if anything is working.

Remove-Repair-Restore

A three-phase framework for gut healing. Remove: eliminate what's damaging the gut (stress, problematic medications, irritating foods, infections). Repair: support gut lining healing with bone broth, fermented foods, and targeted supplements. Restore: rebuild healthy gut bacteria with prebiotic and probiotic foods.

Resistant Hypertension

High blood pressure that doesn't respond adequately to medication. Sleep apnea is one of the most common causes and is dramatically under diagnosed.

Rest-and-Repair Mode (Brake)

The parasympathetic nervous system state that enables healing. Slows heart rate, activates digestion, supports immune function, enables tissue repair, allows deep sleep, and permits nutrient absorption and mineral utilization.

Restless Legs Syndrome (RLS)

A condition characterized by uncomfortable sensations deep in the legs and an overwhelming urge to move them, typically worse at night. Usually caused by low iron affecting dopamine production. Symptoms often resolve when ferritin reaches 75+ ng/mL.

Retest Frequency

How often to check mineral levels once in maintenance. General guidelines: every 1–2 years if maintaining without symptoms; every 6–12 months if managing symptoms with supplements; every 6 months if high-risk.

Rule of Thirds

A method for interpreting lab results beyond simple "normal/abnormal" designations. Bottom third with symptoms = functional deficiency; middle third without symptoms = adequacy; middle third with symptoms = borderline status worth addressing; top third = optimal levels.

S

Safety (Nervous System Definition)

Having the capacity to feel whatever emotions arise—fear, anger, sadness, shame, joy, grief—without judging yourself, pushing them away, or being overwhelmed by them. Not the same as feeling calm all the time or avoiding anything upsetting.

Safety Mode

A nervous system state between Protection and Healing, characterized by stability and some capacity for gradual change. In this state, small, incremental improvements are possible but comprehensive overhauls should be avoided. Represented by the safety icon () in the book's check-ins.

Salty Sweaters

Athletes who lose unusually high amounts of sodium in sweat, visible as salt crusts on skin or clothing. These individuals are at higher risk for electrolyte depletion and require more aggressive replacement.

Seasonal Supplementation

A maintenance approach in which supplements are taken during predictable high-need periods (such as vitamin D in winter or iron around menstruation) rather than year-round.

Selenium

A trace mineral essential for thyroid function, antioxidant defense, and immune health. Brazil nuts are the richest source; 1–2 nuts provide 200% of daily needs. Excessive intake is toxic, so supplementation requires caution. Do not exceed 400 mcg daily.

Serotonin

The "feel good" neurotransmitter targeted by most antidepressants (SSRIs). Zinc is involved in serotonin synthesis. Low zinc can impair serotonin production, potentially reducing antidepressant effectiveness.

Serum Iron

A blood test measuring the amount of iron currently circulating in the blood. One component of a complete iron panel.

Serum Magnesium

The standard magnesium test that measures magnesium floating in blood serum. Less accurate than RBC magnesium because it doesn't reflect intracellular magnesium stores. Request RBC magnesium instead.

Serum Potassium

A blood test measuring potassium levels, included in standard metabolic panels. Optimal range is 4.0–4.5 mEq/L, not just "in range" at 3.5–5.0. Critical for heart rhythm and muscle function.

Serum Zinc

A blood test measuring zinc levels in the blood. Optimal range is 90–120 mcg/dL. Important for immune function, wound healing, and hormonal health.

Sheet Pan Dinner

A meal formula involving protein, cubed potatoes with skin, and vegetables roasted together on a single pan at 425°F. Requires only 5 minutes of prep time with 30 minutes of hands-off baking.

SIBO (Small Intestinal Bacterial Overgrowth)

A condition in which bacteria that normally live in the colon overgrow in the small intestine. Causes gas, bloating, and absorption issues.

Signaling Problem

The phenomenon in which minerals are present in the body but cannot be properly utilized due to insufficient peptide signals directing them. Becomes more common with age as peptide production declines.

Sleep Cascade

The sequence required for sleep: Magnesium → increases GABA (calms brain) → activates parasympathetic nervous system (rest mode) → enables melatonin production → allows sleep. Breaking any link in the chain impairs sleep.

Sports Anemia

Iron deficiency caused by athletic training, resulting from red blood cell destruction through impact, small amounts of gut bleeding during intense exercise, and iron loss in sweat. Common in endurance and female athletes.

Stopping and Assessing

A method for determining whether long-term supplementation is still needed. Choose a calm time, stop one supplement at a time, wait 4–6 weeks, track the specific symptoms that supplement addressed. If symptoms return, restart. If not, remain off unless symptoms return later.

Sublingual

A method of taking supplements (particularly B12) under the tongue, allowing direct absorption into the bloodstream and bypassing digestive absorption issues. Recommended for B12 supplementation, especially for people over 65.

Sunday Prep

A batch-cooking strategy involving approximately 2 hours of weekend preparation (cooking grains and beans, prepping vegetables, hard-boiling eggs, making a sheet pan dinner) to enable quick meal assembly throughout the week.

Survival Mode Problem

The condition in which chronic nervous system activation prevents proper nutrient absorption and utilization, regardless of mineral intake. The body prioritizes immediate threat response over digestion, healing, and mineral metabolism.

Sweat Tax

The mineral losses that occur with every bout of exercise. Average losses per liter of sweat include approximately 800 mg sodium, 200 mg potassium, 10–25 mg magnesium, and 0.5–1 mg zinc. Losses compound over weeks and months of training.

T

T4 to T3 Conversion

The process by which inactive thyroid hormone (T4) is converted to active thyroid hormone (T3). Requires selenium and zinc. Impaired conversion can cause thyroid symptoms despite "normal" TSH.

Thiazide Diuretics

Blood pressure medications such as hydrochlorothiazide and chlorthalidone that deplete potassium and magnesium. Creates a situation where the medication depletes the very minerals needed for cardiovascular health.

Third-Party Testing

Independent laboratory verification that supplements contain what labels claim, in accurate doses, without contamination. Key certifications include USP Verified, NSF Certified, ConsumerLab.com Approved, and Informed-Choice.

Three Core Truths

The book's foundational principles: (1) Your symptoms are real, even when labs are "normal." (2) Food first, supplements second—but supplements aren't cheating. (3) Regulated first, optimized second. Always.

TIBC (Total Iron-Binding Capacity)

A blood test measuring how well the body transports iron. One component of a complete iron panel. Normal range is 250–450 mcg/dL.

Tight Junctions

Connections between cells in the gut lining that control what passes through into the bloodstream. When damaged, these become loose, leading to increased intestinal permeability.

TPO Antibodies (Thyroid Peroxidase Antibodies)

Markers of autoimmune thyroid disease (Hashimoto's). Can be positive while TSH is still normal in early disease. Selenium supplementation reduces these antibodies.

Treatment Dose

The amount of a supplement needed to correct a deficiency, typically higher than the maintenance dose. Examples: Iron treatment 65–130 mg daily vs. maintenance 30–65 mg every other day; Magnesium treatment 400–600 mg daily vs. maintenance 200–300 mg daily.

Treatment-Resistant Depression

Depression that doesn't respond to multiple medication trials. A significant percentage of cases involve undiagnosed nutritional deficiencies (iron, B12, vitamin D, zinc) that impair neurotransmitter production. Testing should occur before the third or fourth medication trial.

Triage System

A conceptual model explaining why hair, skin, and nails show deficiency early. When resources are scarce, the body prioritizes vital organs (heart, brain, liver) first. Hair, skin, and nails are last in line, so they show deficiency before anything else—serving as early warning signals.

Troubleshooting from Regulation

The practice of calming the nervous system before attempting to solve supplement-related problems. Follows the Feel-Pause-Act framework: notice the problem and your nervous system's response, pause before reacting, then make one small adjustment from a calmer place.

U

USP Verified

United States Pharmacopeia verification, a third-party testing seal indicating that a supplement has been independently tested for identity, potency, purity, and dissolution.

V

Villi

Millions of tiny finger-like projections lining the small intestine that dramatically increase surface area for nutrient absorption. Can be damaged by various factors including celiac disease, reducing absorption efficiency.

Vitamin D3 (Cholecalciferol)

The form of vitamin D produced by the body from sunlight exposure. More effective than vitamin D2 for raising blood levels. Requires dietary fat for absorption. Optimal blood level is 40–60 ng/mL.

Vitamin K2

A vitamin that works synergistically with vitamin D and calcium to support bone health and proper calcium utilization. Helps direct calcium to bones rather than soft tissues.

W

When to Move On

Indicators that minerals are not the answer to your health concerns: no improvement after 3–4 months of appropriate supplementation, symptoms worsen, lab values don't improve despite consistent supplementation, or you can't tolerate any form of a supplement.

Z

Zinc Carnosine

A specific form of zinc that supports gut lining healing. Typical dose: 75–150 mg daily.

Zinc Picolinate

A well-absorbed form of supplemental zinc. Preferred over zinc oxide, which has poor bioavailability. Should be taken with food to prevent nausea.

INDEX

#

A

B

C

D

E

F

G

H

I

J

K

L

M

N

O

P

R

S

T

U

V

W

Y

Z

ABOUT THE AUTHOR

Joy Stephenson-Laws, JD

Healthcare Attorney • Certified Wellness Coach • Founder, Proactive Health Labs

Joy Stephenson-Laws, JD, is a healthcare attorney with over forty years of experience and a certified wellness coach. She is the founder of Proactive Health Labs, a national nonprofit helping people take charge of their health—especially when doctors can't figure out what's wrong.

Her path to writing about minerals was personal.

Joy grew up on a farm in Jamaica, where she learned early that soil quality determines everything. Plants in poor soil got sick. Animals without the right minerals got weak. She also grew up watching her mother take pills religiously for every ailment—and then take more pills to treat the side effects of those pills. Her mother followed her doctors' advice without question, never educating herself or asking why. She ultimately died from complications of diabetes and hypertension, conditions that might have been managed differently with better information and a more collaborative approach to her care.

Years later, as a healthcare attorney in California, Joy saw the same patterns—in her clients and in herself. Exhausted, anxious, dismissed by doctors who said their labs were "normal." Doing everything right and still feeling terrible. That search for answers—and the lessons from watching her mother—led her to the connection between minerals, stress, and the nervous system. It also convinced her that we must educate ourselves, formulate the right questions, and work with our doctors as partners rather than passive patients. This book is the result.

Through Proactive Health Labs, Joy and her team have published hundreds of evidence-based articles helping people understand their bodies and advocate for their health. That educational library is available free at **phlabs.org/education**.

She first explored this topic in *Minerals: The Forgotten Nutrient*, co-written with three physicians. That book was thorough but technical—written for people who wanted the science. This book is different. It's for the person who's exhausted, foggy, and needs answers they can actually use.

Joy lives in California, where she continues her advocacy work and plays golf—not because she wants to be a golf professional, but because it teaches her to breathe, stay present, and forgive herself when she misses.

Also by Joy Stephenson-Laws

From Chains to Wings: A Poetry Revolution for Healing—which introduced the Notice—Validate—Adjust framework: a practice for recognizing your nervous system's patterns, validating them without judgment, and choosing a small, regulated response. The foundation for the Feel—Pause—Act practice in this book.

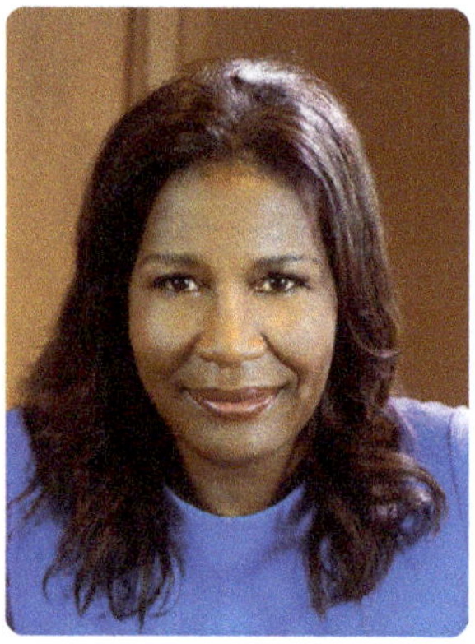

From Chains to Wings: The Workbook—the companion practice guide for building body awareness and nervous system regulation, one pattern at a time.

Secrets That Sparkle (and Secrets That Sting)—a children's book built on a principle that applies at every age: not everything that looks fine on the surface actually is. Some things sparkle. Some things sting. The difference lives in what you feel, not what you're told. That is also the premise of this book.

Minerals: The Forgotten Nutrient—the earlier, more technical exploration of mineral health, co-authored with three physicians, for readers who want the full science.

ACKNOWLEDGMENTS

No book happens alone. This one especially.

First, to my husband Eric—for being fully present with me through every stage of this journey, and for your patience as I navigated mountains of research, often late into the night and early in the morning. Your steady presence made this possible.

To my son Kyle—who taught me what capacity really means. The Protection-Safety-Healing framework exists because of you. You showed me that the same information doesn't land the same way depending on where someone is, and that meeting readers where they are matters more than saying everything at once. This book is gentler and more useful because of what you taught me.

To my family and friends in Jamaica—whose knowledge of the land shaped my roots and my understanding of food as medicine long before I had words for it.

To Dr. Pauline Jose, Dr. Franz Gliederer, and Dr. Monya De—the first physicians I brought into Proactive Health Labs. Each of you taught me something essential about reading medical research with rigor and discernment. Those lessons are woven throughout these pages.

To everyone who read early drafts and told me the truth about what would resonate and what wouldn't—this book is clearer because of your honesty.

To the people who shared their stories with me over the years—the ones who did everything right and still felt terrible, who were dismissed and gaslit, who kept searching for answers anyway. You're why I wrote this. I hope you see yourselves in these pages.

And to you, the reader. Thank you for trusting me with your time and your health. I don't take that lightly.

This book exists because none of us were meant to figure this out alone.

www.ingramcontent.com/pod-product-compliance
Lightning Source LLC
LaVergne TN
LVHW070831220926
848486LV00030B/270
* 9 7 9 8 9 9 3 9 7 4 0 5 7 *